Adolescents at Clinical High Risk for Psychosis

Springer Nature More Media App

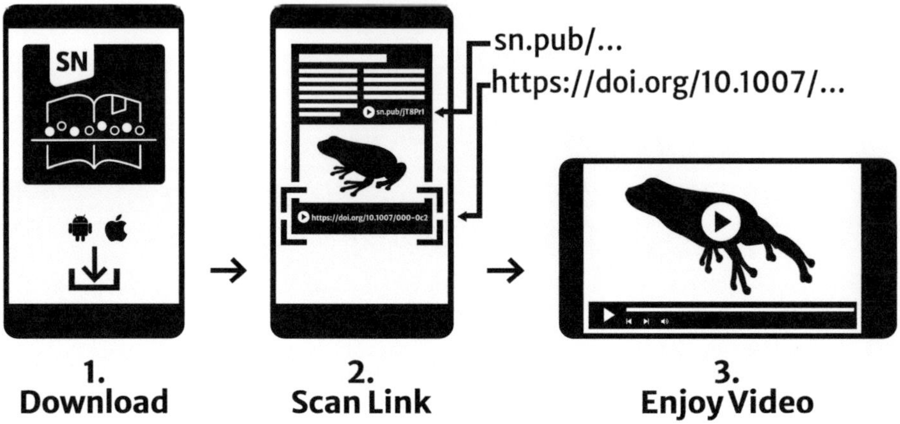

Support: customerservice@springernature.com

Nina Traber-Walker • Maurizia Franscini

Adolescents at Clinical High Risk for Psychosis

Smartphone- App Supported Treatment Approach Robin

Springer

Nina Traber-Walker
University Hospital of Psychiatry Zurich
Department of Child and Adolescent
Psychiatry
Zurich, Switzerland

Maurizia Franscini
University Hospital of Psychiatry Zurich
Department of Child and Adolescent
Psychiatry
Zurich, Switzerland

This work contains media enhancements, which are displayed with a "play" icon. Material in the print book can be viewed on a mobile device by downloading the Springer Nature "More Media" app available in the major app stores. The media enhancements in the online version of the work can be accessed directly by authorized users.

ISBN 978-3-032-10340-6 ISBN 978-3-032-10341-3 (eBook)
https://doi.org/10.1007/978-3-032-10341-3

Jugendliche mit erhöhtem Psychoserisiko - App-unterstützte Behandlung mit dem Therapieprogramm Robin, Springer Berlin, Heidelberg, 2021.

Translation from the German language edition: "Jugendliche mit erhöhtem Psychoserisiko - App-unterstützte Behandlung mit dem Therapieprogramm Robin" by Nina Traber-Walker and Maurizia Franscini, © Springer-Verlag GmbH Deutschland, ein Teil von Springer Nature 2021. Published by Springer Berlin, Heidelberg. All Rights Reserved.

This Springer imprint is published by the registered company Springer Nature Switzerland AG
The registered company address is: Gewerbestrasse 11, 6330 Cham, Switzerland

Foreword by McGorry

One of the major paradigm shifts in psychiatry in recent years has been the prospective definition and recognition of an initial stage of emerging mental illness characterized by subthreshold positive psychotic symptoms and with a clear-cut need for care and impaired functioning. A minority of young people, around 20–30%, who meet this clinical phenotype, which is labeled as the "at risk mental state" or the ultra-high-risk (UHR)/clinical high-risk (CHR) state, progress to fully fledged and sustained psychosis which has been termed "first episode psychosis" (FEP), of which around 60% meet criteria for schizophreniform disorder or schizophrenia. The remainder either recover to a greater or lesser extent, or in too many cases the subthreshold psychotic symptoms persist or the patients develop mood, anxiety, and/or other axis 1 disorders.

While some critics originally alleged that to define, study, and treat people with this phenotype was an overreach and a potentially harmful extension of the boundaries of diagnosis, it has become clear and accepted that with distress and moderately impaired functioning even at this early undifferentiated stage of illness there is an undeniable need for care. The only question, which always had to be resolved through clinical trials, was: what elements and sequences of treatment are appropriate, safe, and effective? The guiding framework for such research has turned out to be the clinical staging model, adapted from other healthcare settings, notably oncology, which determines that the risk/benefit ratio has to be respected and interventions utilized in the earlier stages of treatment for a potentially serious and progressive condition to be safer, and furthermore that treatment should be found to be more effective than in later stages.

There has been a great deal of clinical and biological research in this stage of illness since the 1990s. Several forms of intervention have been studied, and most have been found to be at least partially beneficial and effective. None seems to be superior to the others however, so perhaps it is the case that different people respond to different interventions or there is a general and nonspecific benefit to providing support and care. The psychosocial interventions have generally been versions of CBT, but are often complemented by additional modular features linked to the individual pattern of needs that the patients manifest. Sequences of treatment have also been studied in adaptive trials, which mirror how clinicians tend to behave. A recent sequential adaptive trial of this type deliberately set a high bar for recovery and revealed that current treatments all too often fail to achieve full remission and recovery. So there is much room for improvement and innovation.

This is precisely why this treatment manual and the innovative companion smartphone app Robin Z, written and developed by Nina Traber-Walker and Maurizia Franscini, are such a welcome addition to our range of tools to help these vulnerable young people. The authors are highly experienced clinicians who have worked with this patient population for many years and have developed and manualized a sophisticated and compassionate approach to their psychosocial treatment. The treatment approach is modularized, which is important for what is a heterogeneous clinical syndrome and the associated personal and social needs of the patients. It is backed up by evaluation software Robin View, and the authors have conducted a clinical trial, which is foreshadowing positive results. Their digitally integrated approach is highly congruent with the world of their patients and is achieving high levels of engagement and satisfaction. This work is a significant contribution to this dynamic and cutting-edge field and will be of great value to all clinicians working with this group of vulnerable patients. In the context of the global crisis in youth mental health, it will find a growing audience of clinicians and researchers who are building the new paradigms of early intervention and youth mental health.

Professor Patrick D. McGorry, Professor of Youth Mental Health at the University of Melbourne and Director of Orygen (the National Centre of Excellence in Youth Mental Health), is a leading global expert in early intervention for psychosis and internationally renowned for his pioneering contributions to early detection and prevention strategies in young people's mental health.

Melbourne, Australia Patrick D. McGorry

Foreword by Walitza and Schmidt

The authors, Nina Traber-Walker and Dr. Maurizia Franscini, established the Early Detection and Intervention Service for Psychosis at the Department of Child and Adolescent Psychiatry at the Psychiatric University Hospital Zurich. Inspired by this work, they developed the smartphone app-supported treatment approach Robin for adolescents with clinical high-risk (CHR) symptoms. Psychotic disorders in children and adolescents are serious psychiatric illnesses that often have a prolonged course, leading to multiple psychosocial impairments. Early identification, prevention, and treatment are therefore crucial. However, the nonspecific warning signs of a psychotic disorder only become apparent over a longer period of time. Even young people with milder risk symptoms can experience significant distress, although most will not develop full-blown psychosis.

The present therapy manual is based on evidence-based, multimodal treatment modules that address the complexities of CHR conditions. Drawing on the authors' extensive clinical experience, each chapter offers a practical and accessible approach. The program not only focuses on CHR symptoms but also on common comorbid symptoms such as anxiety, depression, and substance use, as well as psychosocial difficulties. The therapy program is enriched by numerous case examples and practical instructions and explanations of the individual therapy steps. The authors have taken particular care to present the material in a practical way that is accessible to therapists who are new to working with patients in a CHR state, while also serving as a valuable guide for experienced professionals.

To enhance the therapy program for this age group, both authors have developed the smartphone app Robin Z with dedicated effort and by overcoming numerous administrative hurdles. The app has been available free of charge in several languages in the App Store and via Google Play since 2017. The Robin Z app was initially evaluated by patients and clinicians of the Department of Child and Adolescent Psychiatry at the Psychiatric University Hospital Zurich. According to feedback from patients and therapists, adolescent compliance and motivation to actively participate in therapy, for example, by documenting therapy-relevant aspects of their daily lives, have increased. The app is user-friendly and appeals to young people on an appropriate and contemporary level. Great attention has been paid to data protection. Each chapter of the book includes individual app features such as crisis intervention, a logbook to track mood and symptoms, or coping strategies, and is explained in tutorial videos.

The effectiveness of the therapy manual and app is currently being systematically evaluated in a comprehensive treatment trial compared to the current clinical treatment as usual. Initial results confirm the applicability and indicate a high level of acceptance and satisfaction among adolescents.

We wish you and your patients much therapeutic progress and satisfaction with the manual and Robin Z.

Professor Susanne Walitza, Director of the Department of Child and Adolescent Psychiatry at the University Hospital of Psychiatry Zurich, is a leading international expert in child and adolescent psychiatry, especially in ADHD, anxiety, OCD, and pathological media usage.

Professor Stefanie J. Schmidt, Head of the Division of Clinical Child and Adolescent Psychology at the University of Bern, is a leading expert in the treatment of clinical high-risk (CHR) for psychosis.

Zürich, Switzerland Susanne Walitza
Bern, Switzerland Stefanie J. Schmidt

Acknowledgments

This book would not have been possible in its current form without the tremendous support of several people. First and foremost, we would like to thank our medical clinic director, Susanne Walitza, who suggested writing this book in the first place. She has supported us throughout the entire process, both professionally and emotionally, and has stood by our side from the outset. She proofread and commented on all chapters of the manual, providing suggestions to improve its structure.

We would also like to express our sincere thanks to all our colleagues who contributed to the content of the book: Rahel Ammann, Gregor Berger, Yolanda Blumenthal, Maria Raquel Joris, Sibylle Metzler, Markus Karr, Mariama Soumana, and Nadine Uehlinger.

We would like to express our gratitude to One Over Zero, the software company that developed the app Robin Z and the software Robin View. In particular, we would like to thank Roberto Brega for his support and patience throughout this process. We would also like to thank Tanya Schüle and Mattia Cimino for producing the tutorial videos, Mira Cavalli and Alysha Joy Tiziani for designing the avatars, and Pascal Tresch for creating the symbols used in the app and accompanying worksheets.

This English translation could not have been completed without the help of many colleagues who contributed to translating individual chapters. We would like to thank Rahel Ammann, Kristin Anders, Alison Bates, Claudia Bühlmann, Maria Eleni Dimitriades, Miriam Gerstenberg, Tanya Schüle, Melanie Schori, Eveline Voets, and Rubia Wilks for their valuable assistance in revising the English texts. Special thanks go to Mackenzie Rochelle Wilkinson, who meticulously reviewed the entire manuscript and worksheets, providing invaluable linguistic and editorial feedback. Thanks to her dedication and attention to detail, the English version of this book has been significantly improved.

We would like to take this opportunity to thank our colleagues Miriam Gerstenberg, Sibylle Metzler, Fabian Probst, Hadmut Prün, Markus Karr, Elvira Tini, and Eveline Voets from the early detection and intervention service for their excellent cooperation, professional exchange, and joint development of treatment concepts over the past few years.

The book is largely based on our clinical experience during our early intervention consultation hours. We would like to thank our patients and their parents, from whom we have learned a great deal, and for whose benefit we have written this book.

Finally, we could not have written this book without the emotional support of our husbands, Andrea Cavalli and Philippe Traber. Thank you both very much!

Contents

Introduction

1

Psychotic disorders are severe mental illnesses that typically manifest in late adolescence or early adulthood. These disorders cause significant social and economic challenges, along with a substantial burden for both the individual affected and their family. Psychotic disorders are particularly disruptive for young people, as they occur during a crucial phase of personal, social, and educational development.

Psychotic disorders usually develop over a long period of time. Subtle changes in perception, affect, motivation, cognitive functioning, and social skills often precede the full onset of the illness. Early detection research has focused on these changes. The term clinical high risk (CHR) for psychosis has emerged to describe early, subtle changes in thinking, mood, and perception that are clinically relevant but do not yet meet the criteria for full-blown psychosis. In 2013, the Diagnostic and Statistical Manual of Mental Disorders, Fifth Edition (DSM-5) included the diagnosis of attenuated psychosis syndrome in the main text as a codable diagnosis, "other specified schizophrenia spectrum disorder and other psychotic disorder" (code 298.8).

The following theoretical constructs of CHR criteria have been established in the scientific literature and in clinical practice: the basic symptom model (Schultze-Lutter and Koch 2010) and the ultra-high-risk concept (Miller et al. 2003). The basic symptom criteria focus on subtle, subjectively experienced changes in cognition and perception, whereas the ultra-high risk symptoms are attenuated psychotic symptoms in which the ability for reality testing is still intact.

The percentage of patients with CHR symptoms who actually develop psychosis varies among different studies. Early research suggested high transition rates to psychosis, but recent studies estimate them at around 10% (Paolo Fusar-Poli et al. 2015). Regardless of the predictive power of CHR symptoms, they are associated with clinically relevant distress and loss of functioning. Leading experts in the field of early intervention in psychosis have argued that addressing at-risk symptoms in the help-seeking population is warranted regardless of the risk of

N. Traber-Walker, M. Franscini, *Adolescents at Clinical High Risk for Psychosis*,
https://doi.org/10.1007/978-3-032-10341-3_1

transition to psychosis (e.g., Catalán Alcántara et al. 2021; McGorry et al. 2021; Raballo et al. 2022; Shah et al. 2022; Correll et al. 2024). People with CHR and their caregivers report high levels of distress due to these symptoms. The CHR state is also associated with suicidality, impairment in global functioning, and a decline in quality of life. People with CHR report poorer social relationships and higher rates of loneliness than their healthy peers. In addition, individuals with CHR appear to have poor coping skills, low levels of self-efficacy, and negative metacognitive beliefs similar to those seen in patients with depression or overt psychosis. Recent studies have also shown a high prevalence of psychiatric comorbidity in CHR populations with psychosis risk. Furthermore, the CHR state is associated with long-term consequences, independent of conversion to psychosis. A recent study showed that approximately half of non-transitioned CHR individuals remained functionally impaired and had at least one comorbid disorder at a six-year follow-up (Fusar-Poli et al. 2020). On the other hand, CHR individuals who transitioned to psychosis showed poorer clinical outcomes compared to first-episode psychosis patients without a history of CHR symptoms (Malla et al. 2018). Therefore, current data clearly favor targeting and treating at-risk symptoms in help-seeking individuals.

Although CHR symptoms are common in adolescents and are associated with a significant reduction in functioning in this age group, the evidence base needed to guide effective interventions for adolescents with CHR and even first-episode psychosis is lacking. Most intervention studies in the CHR population have focused on adult patients, with only a few including younger patients. Most of these studies used the same treatment approaches for adults and adolescents. Consequently, there is a lack of research on age-appropriate treatment strategies in this vulnerable age group. The transition from childhood to adulthood is a very complex developmental stage, and age-appropriate intervention strategies are needed. The CHR state can disrupt social and psychological development, such as the achievement of educational goals or the establishment of peer relationships. Therefore, adolescents with CHR require treatment strategies that address the complex symptomatology, distress, and impaired functioning. Furthermore, when focusing on engagement in treatment during the first psychotic episodes, the data show that age-appropriate treatment approaches based on adolescents' specific interests are needed in order to engage younger patients.

Our therapy book has been developed as a result of many years of clinical experience with adolescents who meet the CHR criteria. The manual is based on the recommendations for early intervention in CHR states of psychosis of the European Psychiatric Association (EPA) (Schmidt et al. 2015).

Our integrated treatment program is based on cognitive-behavioral, systemic, and solution-focused therapy concepts. Cognitive remediation is used as a supplemental treatment and focuses on improving cognitive and social skills.

In addition to the treatment manual, there are worksheets that can be worked on directly with the patients. The worksheets are encouraging in character. The worksheet texts are mainly positive and written in a language that young people can easily understand, even without therapeutic guidance.

To support patients in their everyday lives between their therapy sessions, the smartphone application (app) Robin Z has been available in the Apple App Store and Google Play Store since September 2017. The use of digital technologies, such as smartphone applications, in therapy has been highlighted as a key element for the future of mental health care. Especially for younger patients, the so-called "digital natives," smartphone apps offer the possibility for age-adapted therapeutic approaches. While there are an increasing number of smartphone apps for young people in the field of eMental Health, there are hardly any studies on the effectiveness of these apps, and most apps have not been developed by clinical specialists (Grist et al. 2017; Torous et al. 2020; Domhardt et al. 2021; Lehtimaki et al. 2021).

Robin Z is one of the first smartphone applications addressing adolescent patients with CHR- or full-blown-psychotic symptoms developed by clinical experts in early intervention for psychosis. The app provides age-appropriate support between treatment sessions, including psychoeducation, symptom tracking, and coping strategies. It helps users understand their symptoms and manage those symptoms better, offers a crisis plan, and includes medication reminders. The app also promotes positive constructs, such as activity suggestions, personal strengths, and weekly goals, offering support in daily life.

The app is developed as an adjunct to therapy and not a replacement for appropriate medical treatment and management. It is not seen as a medical product according to the Swiss Medical Devices Ordinance Act (MepV). We recommend using the app in combination with psychological treatment.

The app works offline and is not connected to the Internet. Data collected by the app is stored in a private directory. These data are protected by the operating system and are inaccessible to other software on the device. The app does not transfer or store any data on the Internet, and no data is stored outside of its private directory. The app is also password-protected.

In addition to the smartphone app Robin Z, we have developed the evaluation software Robin View, which enables adolescents to send their app data to therapists. The therapists thus receive a graphical representation of the young person's individual data, which can be discussed together during therapy.

In November 2021, we started the clinical implementation of Robin Z in four community-based outpatient services of the Department of Child and Adolescent Psychiatry in Zurich, Switzerland. Therefore, we collected data from 27 adolescent patients and their psychotherapists (N = 15) over a six-week period. They all completed questionnaires on user-friendliness and satisfaction with Robin Z and its associated evaluation software, Robin View. The overall results were very encouraging. This first analysis showed that both clinicians and patients consider the app to be applicable and beneficial in therapy. Twenty-six patients (96%) said they would recommend the app to others. Eighteen patients (70%) stated that their mental health condition had improved through the use of the app. All therapists said that they would recommend Robin Z to other therapists. Fourteen therapists (93%) believed that Robin Z was an enrichment to psychotherapy. Patient and therapist feedback was thoroughly evaluated, leading to targeted revisions of the app.

The clinical effectiveness of our therapeutic approach is being investigated in the comprehensive, prospective, controlled follow-up study ETRo (Evaluation of the treatment approach "Robin") (for more information, see Traber-Walker et al. 2019). Long-term data are not yet available and will be analyzed during the coming year. However, an initial evaluation of the intervention group for feasibility, applicability, and subjective satisfaction showed encouraging results (Traber-Walker et al. 2026). According to our evaluation results, the clinical implementation of the treatment program proved feasible. The intervention was applicable and well accepted. In the satisfaction questionnaires, patients rated both the therapy and the smartphone app Robin Z positively. Pre- and post-treatment comparisons indicate a reduction in CHR symptoms and comorbid diagnoses. In addition, significant increases in functionality, self-efficacy, and quality of life were reported after the intervention.

The therapy program is recommended for patients between 12 and 18 years, although some of the material can be used in therapy for young adults over 18 years. Individual modules can also be used for younger patients.

The treatment approach is modular and individualized. Therefore, the book is structured in such a way that each therapist can choose the content that they find useful for their current work with their patients.

The book opens with two case vignettes—Lucy and Michael, fictional adolescents—exhibiting typical CHR symptoms. The following chapters then include exemplary therapy sessions with the two adolescents.

The manual follows the core principles of psychotherapy, beginning with fundamental aspects such as building a therapeutic alliance, involving family members, and setting treatment goals.

Psychoeducation, symptom management, medication management, and crisis management are then covered. In addition, there are chapters on daily activities, hypothetical reasoning, relaxation exercises, and therapeutic work to promote resources.

A detailed explanation of the diagnostic clarification and assessment of CHR for psychosis has been deliberately omitted, including the diagnostic processes, as this manual is primarily a practical guide to therapy and would go beyond the scope of this book. However, reference is made to the literature on the assessment of early symptoms (see Further Reading).

Each chapter includes an introduction for therapists, practical case examples, references to the Robin Z app (including tutorial videos), and worksheets for patients. Suggested further readings and references are provided at the end of each chapter.

References

Catalán Alcántara A, et al. Annual research review: prevention of psychosis in adolescents-systematic review and meta-analysis of advances in detection prognosis and intervention. J Child Psychol Psychiatry. 2021;62(5):657–73.

Correll CU, et al. Identification and treatment of individuals with childhood-onset and early-onset schizophrenia. Eur Neuropsychopharmacol. 2024;82:57–71.

Domhardt M, et al. Mobile-based interventions for common mental disorders in youth: a systematic evaluation of pediatric health apps. Child Adolesc Psychiatry Ment Health. 2021;15:1–12.

Fusar-Poli P, Cappucciati M, Borgwardt S, Woods SW, Addington J, Nelson B, … McGuire PK. Heterogeneity of psychosis risk within individuals at clinical high risk. JAMA Psychiatry. 2015

Fusar-Poli P, et al. Real-world long-term outcomes in individuals at clinical risk for psychosis: the case for extending duration of care. EClinicalMedicine. 2020;28:100578.

Grist R, et al. Mental health mobile apps for preadolescents and adolescents: a systematic review. J Med Internet Res. 2017;19(5):e176.

Lehtimaki S, et al. Evidence on digital mental health interventions for adolescents and young people: systematic overview. JMIR Mental Health. 2021;8(4):e25847.

Malla A, de Bonneville M, Shah J, Jordan G, Pruessner M, Faridi K, et al. Outcome in patients converting to psychosis following a treated clinical high risk state. Early Interv Psychiatry. 2018;12(4):715–9.

McGorry PD, et al. Intervention strategies for ultra-high risk for psychosis: Progress in delaying the onset and reducing the impact of first-episode psychosis. Schizophr Res. 2021;228:344–56.

Raballo A, et al. Clinical high risk for psychosis in children and adolescents: a meta-analysis of transition prevalences. Schizophr Res. 2022;243:254–61.

Shah JL, et al. Early intervention service systems for youth mental health: integrating pluripotentiality, clinical staging, and transdiagnostic lessons from early psychosis. Lancet Psychiatry. 2022;9(5):413–22.

Torous J, et al. Digital mental health and COVID-19: using technology today to accelerate the curve on access and quality tomorrow. JMIR Mental Health. 2020;7(3):e18848.

Traber-Walker N, Gerstenberg M, Metzler S, Joris MR, Karr M, Studer N, ... Franscini M. Evaluation of the combined treatment approach “robin” (standardized manual and smartphone app) for adolescents at clinical high risk for psychosis. Front Psychiatry. 2019; 10:384.

Traber-Walker N, Bühlmann C, Gerstenberg M, Metzler S, Probst, F, Voets E, ... Franscini M. Treatment approach Robin: clinical applicability of a standardised manual and smartphone app for adolescents at clinical high risk for psychosis. J Psychiatr Res. 2026.

Further Reading

Basic-Symptom-Model

Schultze-Lutter F, Koch E. Schizophrenia proneness instrument: child and youth version (SPI-CY). Fioritiit. 2010; Retrieved from http://www.fioriti.it/libri/pdf/Schultze-LutterSPI-CY_EET.doc%5Cnpapers2://publication/uuid/BEAEDEF6-870C-490B-80CD-750C1D4602BE.

UHR-Konzept

McGlashan T, Walsh B, Woods S. The psychosis-risk syndrome: handbook for diagnosis and follow-up. Oxford University Press; 2010.

Miller TJ, McGlashan TH, Rosen JL, Cadenhead K, Cannon T, Ventura J, et al. Prodromal assessment with the structured interview for prodromal syndromes and the scale of prodromal symptoms: predictive validity, interrater reliability, and training to reliability. Schizophr Bull. 2003;29(4):703–15. https://doi.org/10.1093/oxfordjournals.schbul.a007040.

Guidance European Psychiatric Association (EPA)

Gaebel W, Großimlinghaus I, Kerst A, Cohen Y, Hinsche-Böckenholt A, Johnson B, et al. European Psychiatric Association (EPA) guidance on the quality of eMental health interventions in the treatment of psychotic disorders. Eur Arch Psychiatry Clin Neurosci. 2016;266(2):125–37. https://doi.org/10.1007/s00406-016-0677-6.

Schmidt SJ, Schultze-Lutter F, Schimmelmann BG, Maric NP, Salokangas RKR, Riecher-Rössler A, et al. EPA guidance on the early intervention in clinical high risk states of psychoses. Eur Psychiatry. 2015;30(3):388–404. https://doi.org/10.1016/j.eurpsy.2015.01.013.

Schultze-Lutter F, Schimmelmann BG, Maric NP, Salokangas RKR, Riecher-Rössler A, van der Gaag M, et al. EPA guidance on the early detection of clinical high risk states of psychoses. Eur Psychiatry. 2015;30(3):388–404. https://doi.org/10.1016/j.eurpsy.2015.01.013.

Case Studies

2

The following two case studies illustrate typical symptoms of adolescents with clinical high risk (CHR) seen during consultations at our early intervention center for psychosis.

2.1 Lucy, 15 Years Old, Grammar School Student

Lucy has noticed a change in her well-being over the past few months. No matter how much she sleeps, she is constantly tired. She feels increasingly lethargic and lacks motivation. At home, she often just lies on her bed and stares at the ceiling. Sometimes she lacks the energy required to pick up her mobile phone from the table, even though she feels like chatting or going online. She feels overwhelmed just by walking to her desk and reaching for her mobile phone.

Dancing used to be her great passion, but now she hardly likes to dance and often skips practice. She also finds herself withdrawing from her friends more and more. She believes they would not understand what is going on with her anyway. They have already said that Lucy is always in a bad mood and does not laugh as much as she used to. Lucy herself does not know what is wrong with her; she just feels more and more depressed. Sometimes she cries for no reason. She has good friends and lovely parents, and things are going well at school. Lucy does not necessarily feel sad all the time. It is more of a gray feeling, or that she does not feel anything at all. Sometimes her feelings seem like they're all the same, whether they are positive or negative, and she does not really care about anything anymore. It is this indifference that worries her. She never used to be like that before.

Although Lucy constantly feels tired and lacks energy, she is often still unable to fall asleep at night. Sometimes she lies awake until three or four in the morning and feels even worse the next day. She can no longer concentrate at school, and she feels like she can't get through the day. Sometimes she is so tired that she falls asleep during the day.

N. Traber-Walker, M. Franscini, *Adolescents at Clinical High Risk for Psychosis*,
https://doi.org/10.1007/978-3-032-10341-3_2

There are moments when Lucy has sudden thoughts that feel strange, as if someone outside of her has placed thoughts into her head. Of course, Lucy knows that it is not possible, but it still feels that way. In any case, her thoughts do not really seem to belong to her anymore. Instead, she thinks that others can hear or read her thoughts as if they were able to see inside her head. Lucy recognizes the impossibility of that, but it always seems that way to her in those specific moments, and she is no longer sure whether others can hear or read her thoughts. What if it is possible that someone from the outside is having a say in her thoughts? Afterward, of course, Lucy knows that it is nonsense, and she feels silly for thinking such a thing.

In addition to questioning the source of her thoughts, Lucy has the feeling that she's being watched, as if someone is standing behind her, staring at her. When she turns around, there is never anyone there. Still, the uncomfortable feeling persists.

Lucy occasionally gets the strange feeling that she is no longer herself, that she is watching herself from the outside. Her activities can feel automatic, as if she were a robot. This state of mind is very uncomfortable and seems to come out of nowhere, though it started about a year ago. Her environment and the people around her often feel completely unreal. When that unreal sense occurs, Lucy feels cut off from the rest of the world or that she is living in a film. At times like this, Lucy is afraid of going mad.

In addition, her eyes sometimes play little tricks on her. She suddenly sees objects get bigger or smaller. Sometimes, just for a moment, the wall seems to move, or the table shakes. Lucy knows it is all in her head, but that makes it all the more concerning. The other day, during a lesson at school, she could hear a baby crying. Of course, it is not a baby, she thought. After all, what would a baby be doing at school? She did not dare ask any of her classmates if they had heard the baby, too. If she had, they would have thought she was crazy.

Due to feeling so low, Lucy has started smoking cannabis in the last year. Smoking a joint calms her down, and she can forget all her problems. Sometimes she can even laugh again, and the laughter helps. Meanwhile, Lucy has noticed that her perceptual changes seem to be more frequent under the influence of cannabis.

2.2 Michael, 16 Years Old, Apprentice

Michael was diagnosed with Attention Deficit Hyperactivity Disorder (ADHD) as a child and has been prescribed medication since. However, things haven't been going very well recently. In fact, he has not felt himself for some time. He has noticed serious changes in himself in recent months. His mood, his way of thinking, and his perception have all changed. He has strong mood swings with intense emotions that leave him confused. He lives in extremes. Sometimes he feels very confident, full of energy, and driven. At such times, Michael has many ideas, and he wants to realize them all at once. He talks fast, is driven, and is open to a lot. In these moments, he thinks that life is wonderful. The next moment, however, his mood can suddenly shift, and he feels extremely sad or completely overwhelmed by himself and the world. At such times, he wants to crawl into bed and never get out. During these downward phases, he can't imagine that things will ever be different again. Yet the phases pass, often for no apparent reason. Happy Michael and sad Michael are like two completely different people.

Michael is easily scared now, much more than he used to be. He often feels uncomfortable in the dark and even leaves the light on in order to fall asleep sometimes. Of course, he does not tell anyone about this, as it would be embarrassing. Additionally, he suffers from anxiety attacks out of the blue. His heart seems to beat faster, he feels like he can't breathe, and his stomach feels queasy. His body starts to tremble, and he panics.

For about 6 months now, Michael has been hearing a voice. At first, it was just a murmur, and he did not understand anything it said. Then the voice got clearer. Michael still can't discern whether the voice is male or female, and sometimes that's because it's a babble of voices speaking all at once. Michael knows that the voices are not real, that he is only imagining them. He has noticed that he only hears the voices when he is alone and especially hears them in the evenings.

The voices make insulting comments. They tell him that he is not worth anything, that he is a burden to his family, and sometimes even that it would be better if he were no longer alive.

Michael tries to ignore the voices as best he can, and that often works. Listening to music also helps. It distracts him, and the voices often become less frequent. Still, the voices frighten him a lot, especially as they have become more frequent recently.

Michael is often unable to concentrate. As a student with ADHD, concentrating and focusing were never easy for him. However, with the help of medication, he was able to perform well enough at school. Now, sometimes he can barely read a page out of a book. His memory has also weakened. Even if he manages to concentrate and read through a text, he often does not remember what he has just read afterward.

Overall, his thinking seems to have become impaired and worsened over time, with the first changes starting over a year ago. Sometimes Michael's thinking is slow and sluggish. Then his thoughts seem to speed up again, at speeds so fast that he cannot keep up with them because his thoughts jump from one thing to another. He also has more trouble finding words. In the middle of a conversation, he can no longer think in the simplest terms. They are on the tip of his tongue, but he just can't find them. It even occurs that he does not always understand exactly what others are saying. He takes jokes or ironic comments literally and personally.

Michael has begun to believe that he is not as smart as he used to be. As a result, he worries a lot about his education. What if he does not get his diploma? As little as he can concentrate now, things are not looking good for him to be able to complete his apprenticeship.

Michael has never been the type to care much about cannabis, but he does like alcohol. When he is in one of his euphoric moods, he can drink way too much. He usually drinks with his friends on the weekend. It's not uncommon that, when he wakes up the next day, he can't remember exactly how the evening ended. Recently, however, he has found that the voices become less frequent if he drinks alone during the week. However, that does not always work. The day before yesterday, the voices were particularly bad even while he was drinking.

Getting Started with Therapeutic Counseling

3

3.1 General Recommendations for the First Session

It is recommended that patients should be allowed to choose their seat in the room where they feel most comfortable. Some may prefer to sit by the door, while others might choose to sit with their back to the window. This preference could be linked to paranoid concerns, making it essential for patients to select their own seat in order to create a more relaxed atmosphere. For similar reasons, if there are cameras in a room, it is important to clearly declare that they are switched off.

The technique of "joining" is also recommended when working with patients meeting the clinical high risk (CHR) criteria. Joining involves starting the conversation with a neutral topic to help the patient feel more comfortable and to reduce anxiety. During the first consultation, it has been found useful for the patient and their parents to introduce themselves at the beginning of the conversation. This not only provides key background information but also allows a gradual transition to discussing the presenting problem.

In the initial consultation, it is important to identify the patient's different problem areas. Many therapists may hesitate to ask about psychotic symptoms, but experience shows that patients often feel relieved when such questions are addressed. However, it is important to readdress symptoms that are initially negated in further sessions, as many patients do not feel ready to disclose all their symptoms during the first meeting.

CHR symptoms can cause significant distress and often lead to suicidal thoughts. Therefore, suicidal tendencies and potential danger to others need to be thoroughly assessed during the initial consultation. It is advisable to explore suicidal behavior without parents, as young people often feel uncomfortable discussing it in front of

---

Supplementary Information The online version contains supplementary material available at https://doi.org/10.1007/978-3-032-10341-3_3. The videos can be accessed individually by clicking the DOI link in the accompanying figure caption or by scanning this link with the SN More Media App.

N. Traber-Walker, M. Franscini, *Adolescents at Clinical High Risk for Psychosis*,
https://doi.org/10.1007/978-3-032-10341-3_3

them and might withhold information. Therefore, it is beneficial to divide the initial consultation into three parts: the first with both the parents and the patient, the second with the adolescent alone, and the final part with everyone together again. A summary at the end of the interview is recommended to ensure clarity and understanding.

Investing enough time to explore patients' resources and identify parts of their lives that are still functioning is essential for a successful initial consultation. This approach not only helps patients leave the session feeling more positive and motivated to return but also provides the therapist with valuable insight into potential starting points for therapy.

An example of an initial consultation is provided below.

Example of a Therapeutic Conversation: The Initial Meeting with Lucy and Her Parents

Therapist:	I am really glad that you have all been able to come together today. In this first meeting, we will all talk together at the beginning. After that, Lucy, I'd like to talk to you alone, if that's all right with you and your parents. At age 15, there are often some topics that are easier to discuss privately than in front of your parents. If there's any question you don't feel comfortable answering, that's completely fine. I also want to make it clear that I'm bound by doctor-patient confidentiality. If you tell me something in private, Lucy, I won't tell your parents unless we have agreed differently beforehand. There are a few exceptions—for example, if I think you're at risk of harming yourself or someone else, I have to inform your parents. But I will always tell you first, and we can discuss how to handle it together. Are there any questions? *Lucy and her parents shake their heads.*
Therapist:	All right. To start with, I think it would be helpful if everyone could introduce themselves briefly. Maybe we could start with your parents? Could you share a little about yourself and your family? *The parents nod. The mother starts talking:* "I am Lucy's mum. I studied law, and at the moment I work 80% as a lawyer in a law firm where we are three partners."
Therapist:	That sounds exciting, but I'm sure it's also quite demanding and a lot of work.
Mother:	*(nods)* it is. I spread my 80% workload over five days, so I'm not home too late in the evening, and we can still have dinner together as a family. That's really important to me. Luckily, I have a husband who loves to cook. *Lucy's mother laughs.*
Therapist:	This is a real stroke of luck, you could say. *Turning to the father:* So you're the one who enjoys cooking?
Father:	*(nods)* yes, that's me. Cooking is a great way for me to unwind from the office. I'm an accountant, and I work full-time for an insurance company. Fortunately, I have a short ten-minute walk to work, so I'm often home earlier than my wife, and I cook for the family.
Therapist:	So, family dinners are important to everyone?
All three:	*(nodding)*
Therapist:	*(turning to Lucy)* and who else is in the family?
Lucy:	My sister, Kim. She is 13 and is in her first year at secondary school.
Therapist:	And how do you two get along?
Lucy:	*(shrugs)* Most of the time, we're good. Sometimes she can be annoying.
Parents:	*(laugh)*
Mum:	Kim is very attached to Lucy. Lucy is her role model. It's always been that way. Whatever Lucy does, Kim wants to do it too.

Therapist:	Yes, it can be challenging at times, but it must be nice to be admired like that, right? What does your sister admire you for?
Lucy:	Well, I can do things that she can't do because I'm older.
Therapist:	That's true; it's often like that with older sisters. But at 13, your sister can surely do a lot. It might take a little more to keep her admiration. What is it that she admires about you?
Lucy:	We both dance. She's only been dancing for a year, while I've been doing it for longer. So, of course, I'm much better.
Therapist:	Do you dance? What kind of dance?
Lucy:	Modern. And hip-hop for the last six months.
Therapist:	How often do you practice?
Lucy:	Usually twice a week, but lately I've been skipping a lot because I'm just too tired.
Therapist:	I'd like to come back to your exhaustion later. But first, is there anything else you'd like to share about yourself? Do you have any other hobbies?
Lucy:	I like reading, and I enjoy spending time with my friends.
Therapist:	Do you meet up with your friends often?
Lucy:	I used to almost every day, but recently, not as much. After school, I'm often so exhausted that I just want to go home.
Therapist:	You're at grammar school, which can be tiring. Which grade are you in?
Lucy:	I am in the 4th grade, specializing in Italian.
Therapist:	And how do you like the school?
Lucy:	I don't study as well, I get distracted in class, and I'm not really motivated for school. I also feel very tired most of the time.
Therapist:	I'd like to find out more about this tiredness. Can you describe it a bit more?

3.2 Relationship Establishment and Challenges in Communication with Patients Meeting the CHR Criteria

The core principles of Carl Rogers' Person-Centered Therapy (PCT) are recommended as a basic therapeutic approach. The following sections discuss key aspects of the therapeutic relationship in general, as well as specific considerations when working with patients meeting the CHR criteria.

3.2.1 Authenticity

A genuine and sincere attitude is one of the most important factors in building a strong therapeutic relationship. The choice of language is central to this. It is not advisable to adopt a young person's language or imitate their slang, as young people tend to react critically when adults try to appropriate their vocabulary. Further, therapists should only suggest interventions that they really believe in and can commit to.

Patients with CHR symptoms, particularly those with paranoid thoughts, can be very suspicious. They often observe the therapist's behavior closely, paying particular attention to facial expressions and gestures. This is often the case when the therapist is pretending to be someone else. If the therapist feels uncomfortable in the interaction, it's better to acknowledge this rather than ignore it. Otherwise, the therapist's behavior may seem "strange" to the patient, which can lead to increased distrust, as the patient may suspect that the therapist is withholding something or has hidden motives.

3.2.2 Unconditional Positive Regard

Unconditional positive regard refers to a basic acceptance of a person, regardless of what they say. An appreciative attitude is crucial to establishing a strong therapeutic relationship, especially during the initial contact. The patient's statements should be accepted openly and without judgment. The therapist should inquire with genuine interest and try to understand the patient's perspective. The aim is to engage with the young person's constructs of reality without adopting a corrective stance during the first encounter.

Providing regular positive feedback to the patient is key, especially in family discussions. As a therapist, you are an important role model in demonstrating how to communicate and address behavioral problems in an appreciative way.

When addressing the patient's difficult situation, it should be done with care and appreciation.

It is equally important to give patients a sense of autonomy in the course of their treatment. Minors, in particular, should be recognized as responsible individuals capable of making their own decisions.

3.2.3 Empathy

Empathy, in the sense of understanding the patient's perspective, is particularly important when working with adolescents suffering from CHR symptoms. They often struggle to make sense of their own personal experiences, leading to uncertainty. This makes it even more important for the therapist to respond empathically to their stories and emotions. The therapist should engage with the patient's perception of their reality and meet them where they are in their own experience. For example, the belief that they are being monitored and manipulated by aliens is understandably frightening for the patient, regardless of whether the therapist shares this belief. The therapist's own views (e.g., "there are no aliens") should not be imposed on the patient. Similarly, a lack of insight into symptoms must be approached with empathy and understanding.

3.2.4 Transparency

An attitude of transparency is essential for successful collaboration. Any prior information from previous practitioners or referring specialists should be disclosed. The next steps in assessment and treatment should be openly discussed, and it is important to obtain the patient's active consent to each step. For example, if a neuropsychological assessment is planned, the reasons for this should be explained, and the patient's explicit consent should be requested.

The term "psychosis" should not be avoided. In an initial consultation focused on the early detection of psychosis, it should be stated openly that the aim is to assess CHR symptoms. Most patients referred by an external therapist will already be familiar with the term. Others may have researched their symptoms online and found frightening or discouraging information. During the initial consultation, it is important to explain that depictions of psychosis in movies and fiction do not accurately reflect the clinical reality of the illness. The stereotype of the "psychotic axe murderer" should also be dispelled to reduce any unnecessary anxiety or stigma.

3.2.5 Active Listening

Active listening means being fully engaged while the other person is talking to you. It is listening with the intention of gaining a full comprehension of what the other person is saying, rather than listening in order to respond. Active listening implies listening without judging or jumping to conclusions. As such, it is essential for building trust in the therapeutic relationship and can be particularly helpful in reducing mistrust or skepticism in suspicious patients. Active listening involves the following:

- To remain attentive and focused, to maintain eye contact, and to use non-verbal cues such as nodding to show you are listening.
- To regularly summarize what the patient has said, using the words selected by the patient.
- To ask for confirmation to ensure you have understood them correctly.

3.2.6 Normalizing

A depathologizing approach to CHR symptoms is central and beneficial for patients. In particular, perceptual changes or paranoid symptoms should be presented as part of the normal human experience. For example, while over 10% of people experience such phenomena at some point in their lives, the lifetime prevalence of developing a psychotic disorder is only 1%. It's important to help young people understand that their symptoms are common among others of their age. This can be conveyed by framing questions such as "Many young people who come here mention that they sometimes feel like they're being watched, even when no one is around. Has this ever happened to you?"

In addition, references to dreams, age-appropriate magical thinking in childhood, or even drug-related experiences can help patients understand that these unusual experiences can happen to anyone under certain circumstances.

However, it is important to ensure that normalizing these symptoms does not come across as trivializing their suffering.

3.2.7 Optimistic Attitude to Change

Most patients experience high levels of distress due to their CHR symptoms. Statements such as "If this doesn't stop, I don't want to live anymore" are not uncommon. This makes it all the more important for the therapist to maintain an optimistic attitude and to emphasize that these symptoms are treatable. The therapist should reassure the patient that strategies can be learned to cope better with CHR symptoms. In cases of severe distress and perceived functional impairment, the possibility of medication should be introduced as part of the treatment plan.

Many patients feel powerless and overwhelmed by their symptoms. It is important to offer a positive perspective. The worksheets provided in Chap. 4 can be helpful in this regard. For example, introducing the concept of "CHR for psychosis" can be reassuring for both patients and parents, helping them to understand that the symptoms are treatable and that, although this is a very difficult period, it is one that can be overcome. Questions about prognosis are often raised at the first consultation. It is important to reply honestly that the prognosis is uncertain. However, it is also important to reassure the patient that they are not currently experiencing psychosis, but rather psychosis-related CHR symptoms. It is important to clarify that being at CHR for psychosis does not necessarily mean developing psychosis, as the transition rates are low. According to current research, the transition rate is around 10%. An important reason for this low transition rate is the therapeutic treatment of CHR symptoms.

The overall essential experience from our clinical practice is that all patients make progress. The progress is highly individual and sometimes small—so small that it might not be noticed by patients or their environment. It is therefore important to consistently emphasize progress to both patients and their caregivers. In the sense of therapeutic optimism, questions about symptom-free moments, coping strategies, and positive changes achieved should be asked at the first consultation. Most patients only seek consultation after living with symptoms for a long period of time, sometimes months or even years. During this time, they have often developed coping strategies for managing their symptoms, which should be explored and acknowledged during the consultation.

3.2.8 Dealing with Mistrust and Delusional Thinking

As mentioned earlier, adolescents with CHR symptoms can be very distrustful and suspicious in therapy. The therapist's primary challenge is to withstand this distrust. An open and transparent attitude towards the patient can help to overcome this suspicion.

During the initial consultation, most patients are not ready to question their delusional thoughts. Rather than doubting their statements, the therapist should aim to gain as full an understanding as possible of the patient's world of experience through active questioning. Abrupt interventions such as "It's not real, you're imagining it" risk losing the patient's commitment from the start. Once a therapeutic relationship has been established, the therapist can begin to challenge the patient's unfavorable beliefs through hypothetical reasoning.

When asked for an opinion on the patient's thoughts and theories, it is advisable for the therapist to use "I-statements," such as:

"I've never heard anything like it, and I know of no evidence to support your assumption."
"I don't think so."
"I can't imagine that."

These responses can help the patient feel that their concerns are being taken seriously. Statements such as "That's certainly not the case" or "It's impossible" can come across as dismissive and fail to validate the patient's concerns. The therapist should not automatically assume that everything the patient says is delusional. Even obviously paranoid patients may have valid reasons for feeling watched, bullied, or persecuted.

If the thoughts are not dangerous to the patient or others, the assessment can be continued in an outpatient setting. Immediate hospitalization should only be considered in cases of severe delusional thinking that endangers the patient or others. However, this is relatively rare when working with patients meeting the CHR criteria, as they are generally able to reflect and check their reality.

3.2.9 Dealing with Formal Thought Disturbances

Impairment in formal thinking can already be present in a patient meeting the CHR criteria and may complicate the conversation. Commonly observed thinking difficulties include concentration problems, thought blocking, poor memory, and incoherent, illogical, or slow speech. Structuring the conversation can be particularly helpful in these situations. To facilitate communication, long and complicated questions or sentences should be avoided, and technical jargon should be minimized in favor of simple, direct language. Offering short breaks and using visualization aids, such as a timeline (see the related worksheet), can also be helpful in recording symptoms and events. Taking brief notes of what the patient has said can help categorize their statements accurately. The therapist should regularly summarize the patient's comments and verify their understanding by asking for confirmation. If the patient rambles, it is important to return to the main point.

3.3 Involvement of the Family in the Assessment and Therapy

It is essential to involve the patient's family in the treatment process as soon as possible. In everyday clinical practice, inviting parents to the initial consultation and beginning discussions together has proven effective.

During this session, parents should be asked detailed questions about their observations regarding their child's symptoms, such as:

- What differences have you noticed in the behavior of your child?
- When did you first notice these changes?
- In what areas have you perceived impairment?
- Have you noticed any particular symptoms?

Therapists should then explore the parents' hypotheses and explanatory models regarding their child's symptoms. Psychotic symptoms must always be understood in the context of family dynamics, including religious and cultural backgrounds. For example, if the family collectively believes in ghosts, it is not unlikely that the child might have conversations with ghostly beings.

Most parents feel confused by their child's CHR symptoms. They observe changes in behavior but often struggle to interpret them or know how to respond. Therapists should encourage parents to continue to see themselves as experts on their children while providing support in relation to the symptom. It is therefore helpful to give parents space to express their fears and questions about the symptoms. Some may find it difficult to express these concerns in family meetings, as they may want to protect their child from distress. In such cases, it may be beneficial to meet parents alone.

After the diagnostic phase, a comprehensive psychoeducational session should be conducted with the entire family. Historically, various theories have identified parents, particularly mothers, as the cause of psychotic disorders. In particular, the term "schizophrenic mother" has long shaped the attitudes of many psychologists and psychiatrists involved in the treatment of psychosis. Even today, parents often feel guilty and stigmatized about their children's mental health problems. This makes it all the more important to provide parents with thorough psychoeducation about psychosis and its etiology (see also the next chapter).

Identifying and acknowledging family factors contributing to the development or maintenance of symptoms is crucial, while also focusing on the resources and opportunities for positive change.

The worksheet "How Did My Problems Start?" can be used along with the worksheet "How Did My Problems Arise?" to create an individualized picture of the disorder within the family. Additionally, the worksheet "What Can We Do About It?" can facilitate a dialogue about the actions each family member can take to improve the situation.

The psychological well-being of the parents is an important factor in the prognosis. If parents need more support than is provided by parental guidance, therapists should encourage them to seek therapeutic help independently.

Involving siblings is another important aspect of family involvement. Experience in everyday therapeutic practice suggests that siblings are often overlooked. They should also be offered the opportunity to voice their concerns and questions. In many families, symptoms go unspoken, and siblings are unaware of their sister's or brother's situation. This is often because they do not want to burden their sibling with the problem and protect them from it. In the majority of cases, however, the sibling realizes that something is wrong and is concerned. Clarifying conversations can be very helpful.

Younger siblings, in particular, may react to their sibling's illness with symptoms of their own, sometimes in an attempt to get parental attention.

It is important to communicate with younger children in a child-friendly manner, explaining that their sibling is having problems at the moment and that their parents need to provide a little more attention, but that they are receiving medical treatment and their siblings do not need to worry.

It is advisable to reassure the siblings that they are not responsible for their brother or sister's recovery and that they will be offered help with therapy. Furthermore, the sibling relationship can be an enormous resource for positive treatment outcomes, especially for patients with severe social withdrawal, as siblings are often the only peers with whom they interact.

Even when parental behavior is seen as problematic, it is still important to maintain a respectful and transparent attitude towards parents. Especially when the therapist identifies family dynamics as contributing to the symptoms, successful treatment depends on good cooperation with the parents.

The therapist should try to remember that parents fundamentally want what is best for their children. All parents want to be good parents. The definition of what is 'best' for the child can vary widely and is subjective; it is not the role of the therapist to judge or completely change parenting.

- During initial meetings, adopting a solution-oriented attitude and framing questions positively can be particularly beneficial. Parents should be encouraged to discuss their children's strengths and resources, which has several benefits.
- Most parents appreciate the opportunity to talk about their children's positive attributes. Therefore, asking about strengths is a good way to build rapport and can help create a positive and comfortable atmosphere during the conversation.
- The therapist gains insights into the patient's resources and learns what aspects of family life are functioning well, providing essential information on which the therapeutic interventions can be built.
- Hearing positive feedback from their parents can have a profoundly uplifting effect on young people and facilitate change.

In cases where parents struggle to express positive sentiments about their children, therapists should remain persistent and continue to prompt questions, such as:

- What do you particularly appreciate about your child?
- What character traits do you admire about your child?
- What is your child better at than others?
- Does your child have special skills?
- What positive aspects of family life do you recognize?
- Can you think of a recent moment that was particularly good?

3.4 How to Set Goals for Therapy

3.4.1 Therapy Goals

The treatment targets should be established at the beginning of therapy. What does the patient expect from the treatment? Are these expectations realistic, and how can they be met? Are there any barriers to achieving the treatment targets? In addition, what are the expectations of the patient's family and the wider community?

It is beneficial to agree with the patient on the specific, realistic goals that they would like to achieve through therapy. The worksheet "Therapy Goals" can be used for this purpose, which is structured for up to three goals. Of course, fewer goals can be addressed, and in some cases, more can be identified. However, it is not advisable to focus on too many aims at once. It is important to discuss how the patient intends to achieve their goals and how they will recognize their progress.

For certain goals, a more detailed plan for achieving them may be helpful. This plan should be written down with the use of the second worksheet, "How Will I Achieve My Therapy Goal?" Achieving therapy goals will inevitably impact the patient's life. It's essential to discuss these potential effects while setting goals. This includes considering not only how the patient will be affected but also the impact on the entire family system.

Some key questions to consider include:

- How will achieving this goal change the patient's life? What will be different?
- What will improve, and what challenges might arise?
- How will the family react to the patient achieving their goals? What specific impact will this have on each family member? Is there anyone in the family who might oppose the goal?
- How will achieving the goal affect the patient's relationships with peers?
- How might the patient's partner react?
- Are there any implications for the patient's education or career if the goal is achieved?

These questions are also crucial for the therapist to consider. Sometimes, there are underlying reasons why patients may hesitate or resist achieving their goals. They may show increased symptoms as a way of avoiding success in therapy.

The patient's therapy goals should be discussed with the parents in order to obtain their agreement and support in working on them. The worksheet "Family Goals" can help guide this process. Family goals may be different from individual therapy goals, but if these goals are conflicting or contradictory, this needs to be disclosed and discussed during the family meetings to ensure a collaborative approach.

3.4.2 Weekly Goals

The worksheet "Weekly Goals" is designed to help patients set smaller, achievable objectives each week. There's a double aim: to encourage daily activation and to provide the patient with a sense of accomplishment. During the therapy session, the therapist and patient work together to identify up to three goals that the patient would like to achieve in the coming week. These goals should be realistic and achievable. For example, a goal such as "I will study for two hours every day from now on" is unrealistic if the patient has done little or no schoolwork recently. A more achievable goal might be "I will study for at least 30 minutes on Monday and Wednesday, and once on the weekend." Setting achievable goals increases the likelihood of success and helps build motivation to keep going.

Weekly Goals

The patients can set both long-term and short-term goals under "Weekly Goals," similar to the worksheet. Once a goal is achieved, it can be saved as an achieved goal. Furthermore, in the function "Logbook," the user can mark the achieved goals in each entry.

The Robin View evaluation software provides the therapist with a graphical overview of which goals are still open and which have already been achieved.

Tutorial video 4 "**Weekly Goals**" (Fig. 3.1) explains how to use the weekly goals in the therapy session.

It is important that weekly goals encompass more than just school or work. Other parts of life should also be included when setting weekly goals. A well-rounded target might be "I will arrange to meet someone at least once a week."

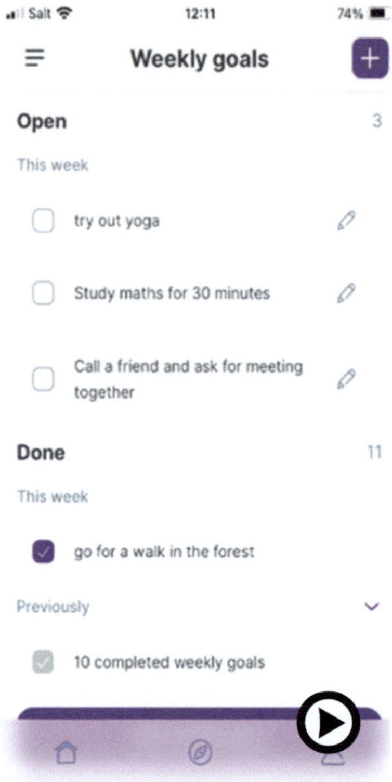

Fig. 3.1 Tutorial video "Weekly goals" (▶ https://doi.org/10.1007/000-k5d)

Therapeutic Conversation with Michael

Michael:	I want to catch up on all the gaps at school.
Therapist:	That's a pretty ambitious goal. Do you think it is realistic to accomplish that in just one week?
Michael:	I have to. There are only two months left until the summer break, and I really want to improve my grades.
Therapist:	That's understandable, and I think it's still a very high target. You're expecting a lot from yourself. I don't think it's possible to catch up on everything you've missed in just one week.
Michael:	What should I do then?
Therapist:	Maybe you don't need to catch up on everything right away. In which subjects would you most like to improve?
Michael:	Chemistry, physics, and French.
Therapist:	That's three subjects.
Michael:	Yes, I'm failing all three subjects.
Therapist:	How many subjects are you allowed to fail?
Michael:	Two.
Therapist:	So if you improve in just one of them, that would be enough to pass the year.
Michael:	Yes, that's true. But I would like to do better in all of them.

Therapist:	I want to remind you that you're going through a difficult time. Maybe this is the time to be selective about where you can do your best. In which of the three subjects would you most like to improve?
Michael:	Chemistry.
Therapist:	So maybe a weekly goal could be to study chemistry?
Michael:	Yes, at least one hour a day.
Therapist:	Is that realistic? Outside of work, one hour a day just for chemistry?
Michael:	No, not really.
Therapist:	How much have you done in chemistry so far?
Michael:	Almost nothing.
Therapist:	Then studying for an hour twice a week would be a real improvement.
Michael:	Yes, it would be.
Therapist:	Can you manage it?
Michael:	I think so.
Therapist:	Great, your first goal for next week is to study chemistry for at least one hour on two different days. Write down the days on which you plan to do this. What would be your second goal?
Michael:	I also need to improve my French.
Therapist:	How about this: You could learn three new French words every day on the train during your commute.
Michael:	Only three?
Therapist:	How many new words have you learned a day so far?
Michael:	None ...
Therapist:	So three a day would be a great improvement.
Michael:	So my third goal is physics.
Therapist:	How about focusing on something that benefits you instead? Like taking some time out every day to do something positive.
Michael:	I don't know if I can do that. With work and school... I'm often too tired to do anything when I get home. And then I have to study.
Therapist:	Do you study when you get home?
Michael:	I should, but I often find it hard to concentrate. Then I end up gaming or going online.
Therapist:	What would you do if you didn't have to study?
Michael:	Maybe go out and play football with my friends in the neighborhood.
Therapist:	What if one of your goals was to play football with your friends for at least an hour, at least once a week in the evening? Would that be good for you?
Michael:	Oh yes. I would get to be outside, play football, exercise, and hang out with my friends. But what about school?
Therapist:	Don't you think it might be easier to study one night, knowing that you don't have to do anything the next day and that you can play football?
Michael:	I think so.

3.5 Worksheets

The following worksheets (Fig. 3.2) belong to this chapter and can be downloaded online as part of the electronic version:

- Worksheet 5 "How Did My Problems Start?"
- Worksheet 6 "What Can I Do About It?"
- Worksheet 7 "What Can We Do About It?"

How Did my Problems Start?

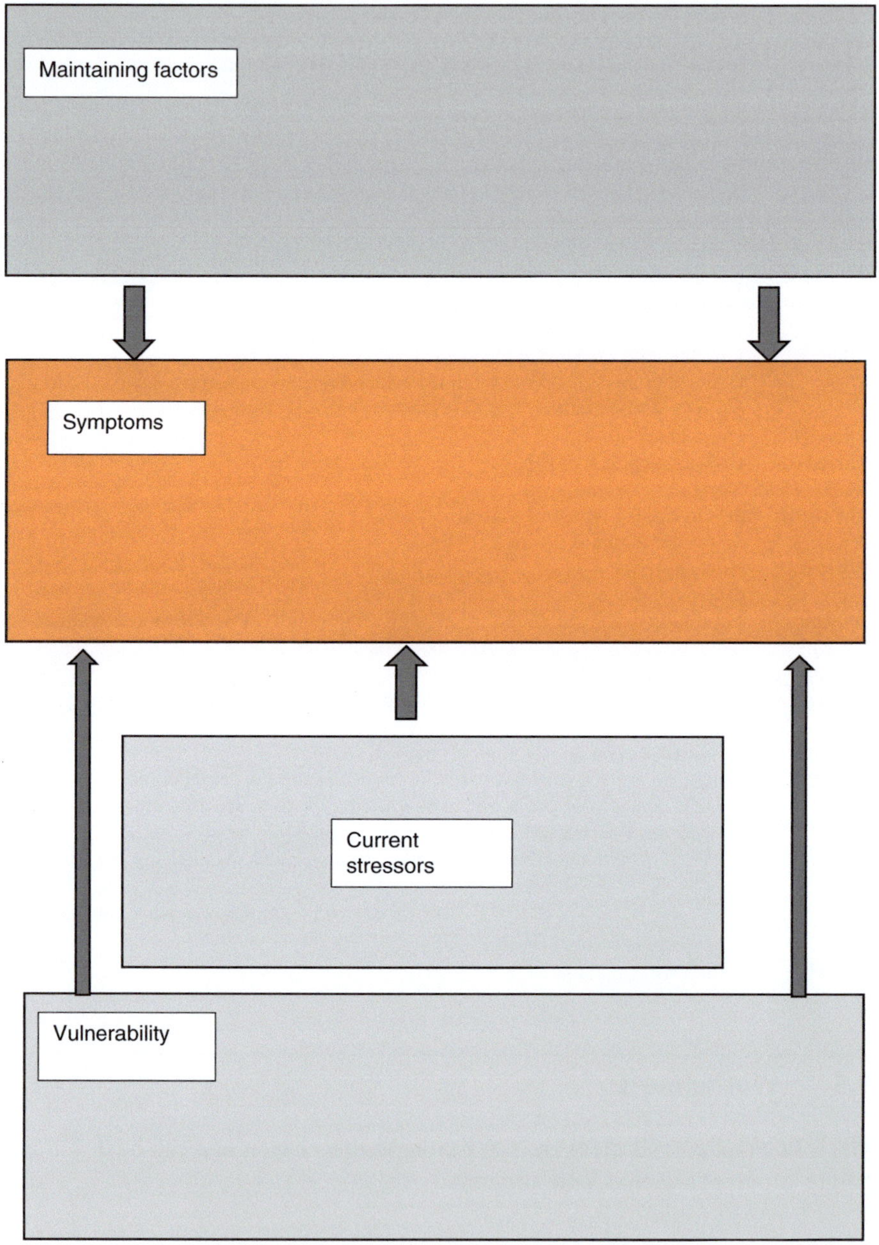

Fig. 3.2 Worksheet 5 to Worksheet 12

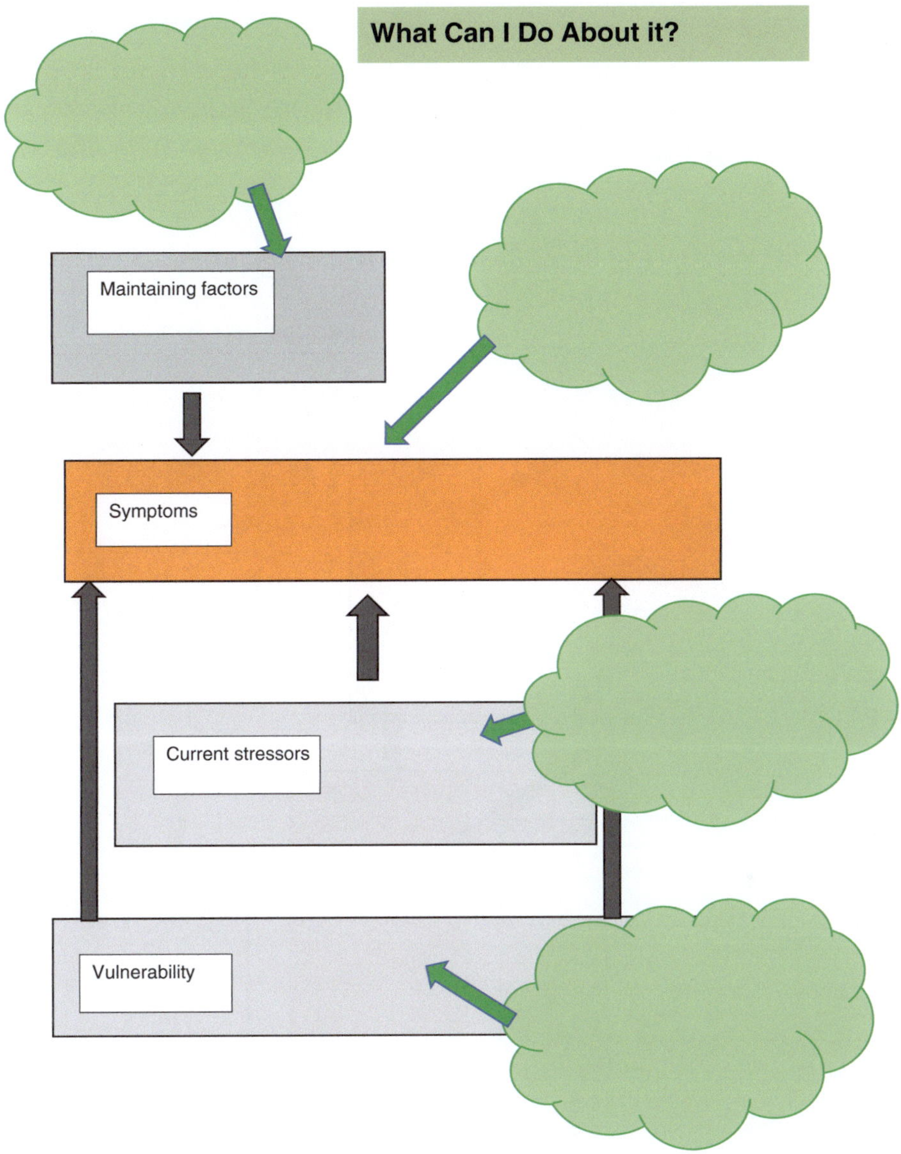

Fig. 3.2 (continued)

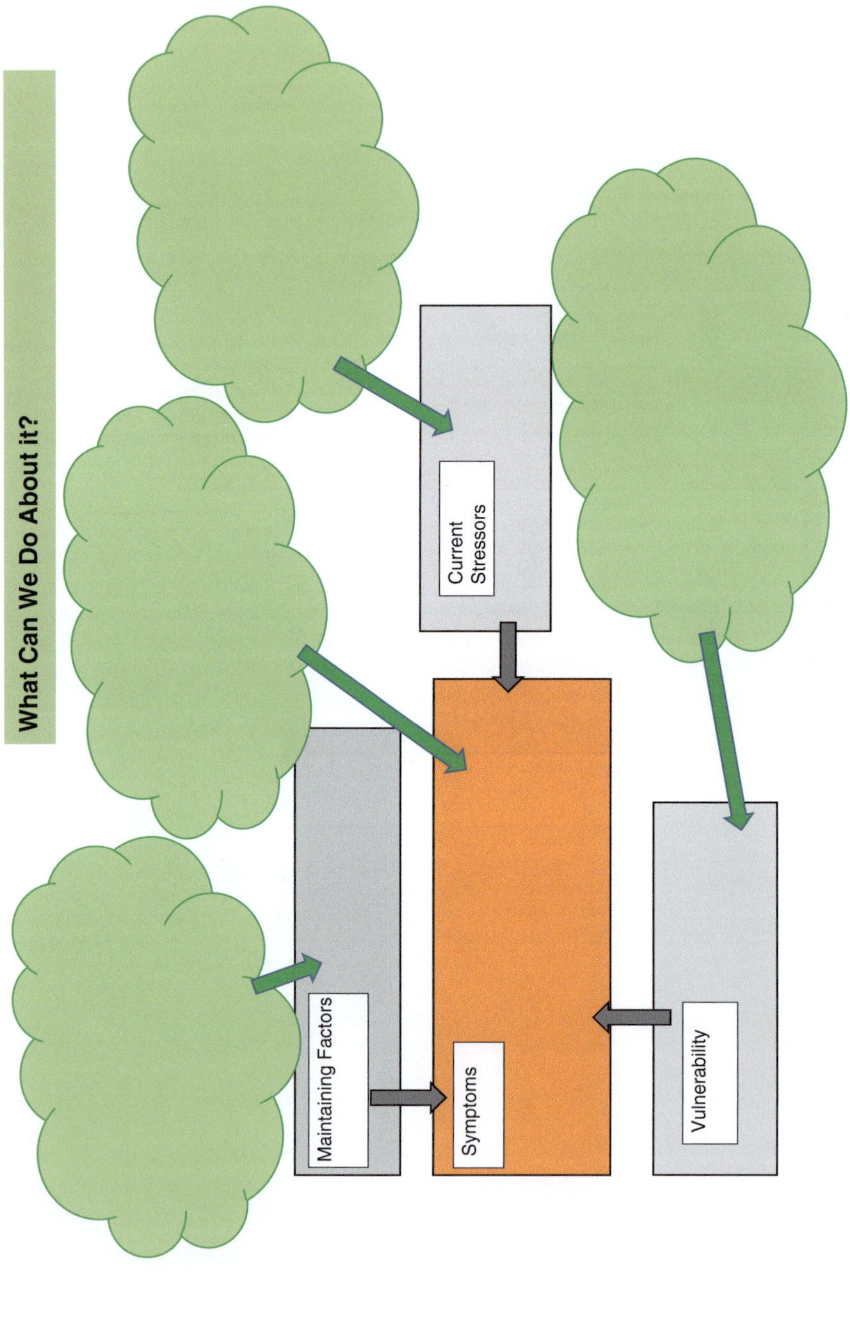

Fig. 3.2 (continued)

Family Goals

Goal

How can the goal be achieved?

Who?	What?	With what resources?

How will we know when the goal has been achieved?

Fig. 3.2 (continued)

Therapy Goals

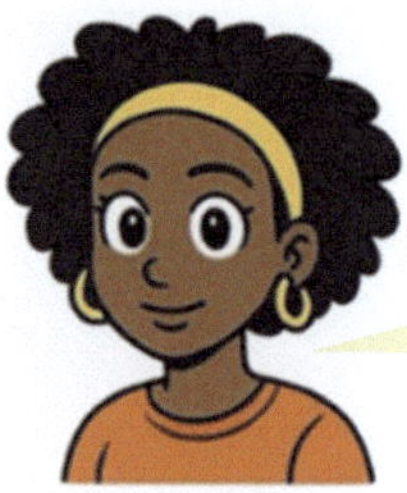

Choose three goals for your therapy. Things you would like to achieve. For example, to develop strategies for dealing with symptoms or to start seeing friends more often.

1. Goal:

How do you know that the goal has been achieved?

2. Goal:

How do you know that the goal has been achieved?

3. Goal:

How do you know that the goal has been achieved?

Fig. 3.2 (continued)

How Do I Achieve My Goal?

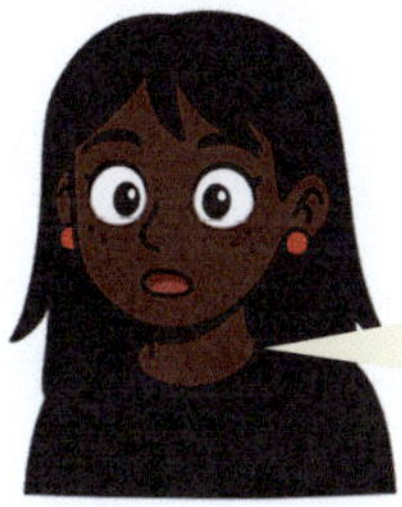

Create a concrete plan with your therapist for achieving your goal.

My goal is:

What exactly will be different once I have reached my goal?

By when do I want to achieve my goal?

What is the first step?

What actions can I take to achieve my goal?

Which of my strengths will help me achieve my goal?

How can therapy support me?

Who in my life could help me achieve my goal?

Fig. 3.2 (continued)

Goal Achievement

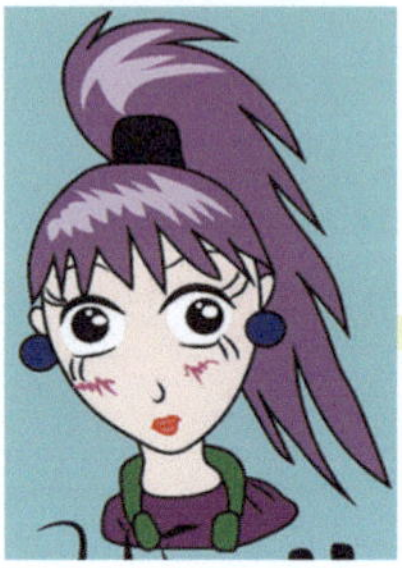

What are your current therapy goals? What have you already achieved? Use a scale to assess where you currently stand.

1. Goal:

Start → Finish

What have you achieved so far?

What is missing?

What would be the next step?

Fig. 3.2 (continued)

2. Goal:

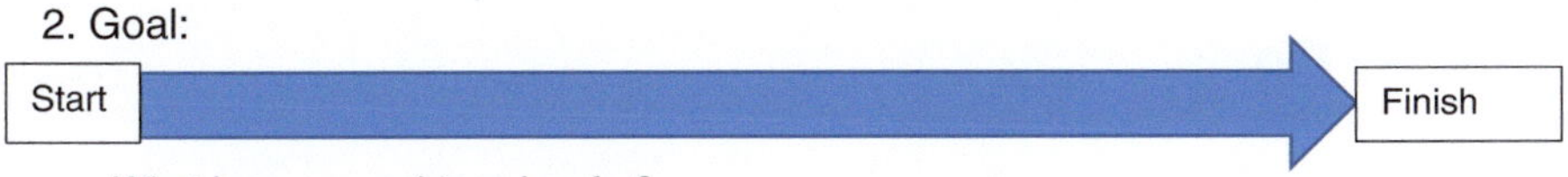

What have you achieved so far?

What is missing?

What would be the next step?

3. Goal:

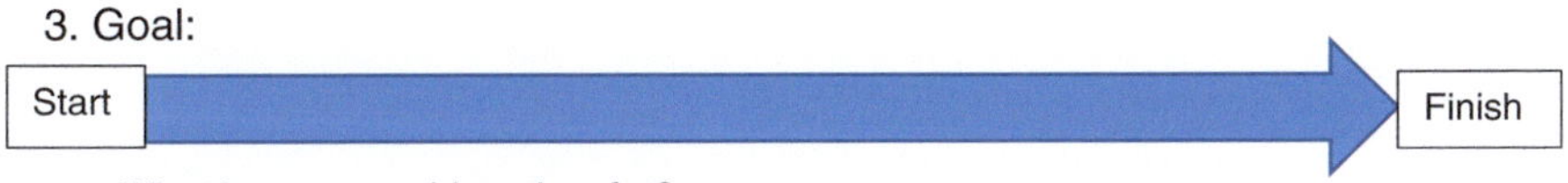

What have you achieved so far?

What is missing?

What would be the next step?

Fig. 3.2 (continued)

Weekly Goals

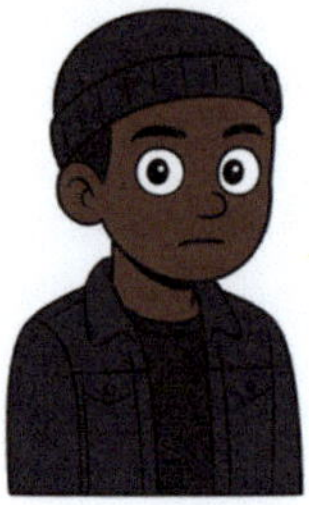

Set three goals for this week. Think of things you would like to do this week. For example, start reading a certain book, or tidy up your room.

1. Goal

Made it:□

2. Goal

Made it:□

3. Goal

Made it:□

Fig. 3.2 (continued)

- Worksheet 8 "Family Goals."
- Worksheet 9 "Therapy Goals."
- Worksheet 10 "How Do I Achieve My Goal?"
- Worksheet 11 "Goal Achievement."
- Worksheet 12 "Weekly Goals."

Further Reading

Rogers C. Client-centered therapy. new ed. Hachette UK; 2012.

4 Psychoeducation

Comprehensive psychoeducation on the concept of CHR for psychosis is an important component in the treatment of patients with CHR symptoms. Not only adolescents themselves, but also their relatives should be informed in detail about the topic.

Comprehensive psychoeducation includes:

- Introduction of the term "psychosis," emphasizing that psychosis is a temporary condition.
- Introduction to the concept of "CHR for psychosis".
- Explanation of the Vulnerability-Stress Model.
- Creation of an individual etiological model of the symptomatology.
- Information about the effects of substance use (see the section on substance use in Chap. 5).
- Information about the treatment options.

Relatives and patients react very differently to the information associated with the risk of psychosis. Some react with great concern; others suppress what they have heard. Our experience is that neither overconcern nor understatement is helpful in this context. In family discussions, it is particularly important to reach a consensus that the current symptoms should be treated. Regardless of whether the criteria for psychosis are met or not, if the patient suffers from perceptual disturbances or social withdrawal due to diffuse delusional fears, it is important to initiate therapeutic steps and support the patient in dealing with them.

Supplementary Information The online version contains supplementary material available at https://doi.org/10.1007/978-3-032-10341-3_4. The videos can be accessed individually by clicking the DOI link in the accompanying figure caption or by scanning this link with the SN More Media App.

N. Traber-Walker, M. Franscini, *Adolescents at Clinical High Risk for Psychosis*,
https://doi.org/10.1007/978-3-032-10341-3_4

4.1 What Is Psychosis?

What actually is psychosis? Psychosis or schizophrenia? Which term should be used?

We use the term psychosis as it covers all types of psychotic disorders. Psychosis is a temporary condition characterized by a disturbance in the individual's perception of reality. It is associated with temporary changes in affect, drive, thoughts, and perceptions. The worksheet "What is Psychosis?" can be used to show examples of each of these categories. Affect and drive are grouped together on the worksheet under the term "mood," as the terms "affect" and "drive" are often less understandable to both patients and parents. Most non-experts, on the other hand, immediately understand what is meant by the term 'mood.' The three categories of mood, thought, and perception are represented as overlapping circles to show that it is not always possible to clearly distinguish between them. Thus, certain CHR symptoms may affect thought and perception as well as affect and drive.

There is no standard psychosis or set of symptoms that must always be present in psychosis. Therefore, psychosis cannot be considered a homogeneous medical condition. Every patient's symptoms are individual. Even patients who experience several psychotic episodes may not necessarily experience the same symptoms during each episode.

Psychoeducation, therefore, requires personalization. This information should be tailored to the patient's needs. It can be helpful to mention both existing and non-existing symptoms of the patient. However, it is important to consider carefully whether mentioning potential symptoms will be more distressing or reassuring for the patient concerned.

4.2 What Does an Increased Risk Mean?

Risk symptoms are impairments in perception, thinking, affect, and drive that do not meet the qualitative criteria for psychosis. In contrast to manifest psychosis, patients who meet the CHR criteria still have the capacity for reality testing. As far as the long-term outcome of the CHR condition is concerned, references can be made to the state of recent research. Currently, a low transition rate (approximately 10%) is assumed for adolescents with CHR symptoms, though previous studies have shown higher rates. One hypothesis for the current lower number of transitions is that early symptoms are now better recognized and treated appropriately. The worksheet "Progression of CHR Symptoms" can be used to visualize the potential development of symptoms and possible remission over time. However, the focus should be on a potentially positive prognosis, especially in view of the current research regarding only a 10% transition rate. There are several reasons why describing a possible positive outcome is important for further treatment. Firstly, a more confident attitude can be achieved in young people and their families. Secondly, patients feel more empowered and less dominated by their symptoms. Finally, treatment motivation is increased when patients can see the potential for recovery.

Psychoeducation is also very important with regard to the individual symptoms; this is discussed in more detail in Chap. 5. Patients can also be given the worksheets on the respective symptoms.

4.3 Vulnerability-Stress Model: How Does Psychosis Develop?

Zubin and Spring (1977) developed the Vulnerability-Stress Model, which is also suitable as an explanatory model for patients in psychoeducation. The Vulnerability-Stress Model is based on an individual's vulnerability. Vulnerability factors include genetic components, pre- and perinatal damage, birth complications, or viral infections in childhood. In addition to biological influences, other factors may contribute to increased vulnerability, such as traumatic childhood experiences, atypical parental situations, or comorbid disorders. According to the model, psychotic symptoms do not arise as a result of increased vulnerability but only in the context of experienced stress. This may be a single stressful experience; however, often it is a chronic stressor that has been present over a period of time. Whether a situation is experienced as stressful is subjective. A difficult situation is perceived as stressful if the person does not have sufficient coping strategies and is no longer able to deal with the situation. Therefore, it is important to emphasize the aspect of subjectively experienced stress when explaining the vulnerability stress model.

Regardless, we can learn to deal with stressful situations more effectively. It is important to remember that it is not only negative events that can cause stress. Positive stressors, such as an exciting trip or falling in love, can also trigger psychotic symptoms.

It is important to go into detail about the individual vulnerability and stress factors of young people and then to create an individual explanatory model. The worksheet "How Did My Problems Arise?" can be used for this purpose. In addition to individual vulnerability factors and triggering events, it also lists factors that sustain the problem, such as dysfunctional thought patterns or personality traits. As contributing factors can be difficult to influence, the second step is to look for coping strategies to deal with vulnerability factors, sustaining factors, and stressful events. These can be summarized on the worksheet "What Can I Do About It?" The worksheet "What Can We Do About It?" is intended for family meetings.

4.4 Worksheets

The following worksheets (Fig. 4.1) belong to this chapter and are available online for download in the context of the electronic chapter:

- Worksheet 1 "What Is a Psychosis?"
- Worksheet 2 "How Does Psychosis Develop?"
- Worksheet 3 "What Causes Psychosis?"
- Worksheet 4 "How Did My Problems Start?"
- Worksheet 5 "What Can I Do About Iit?"
- Worksheet 6 "What Can We Do About Iit?"

What Is a Psychosis?

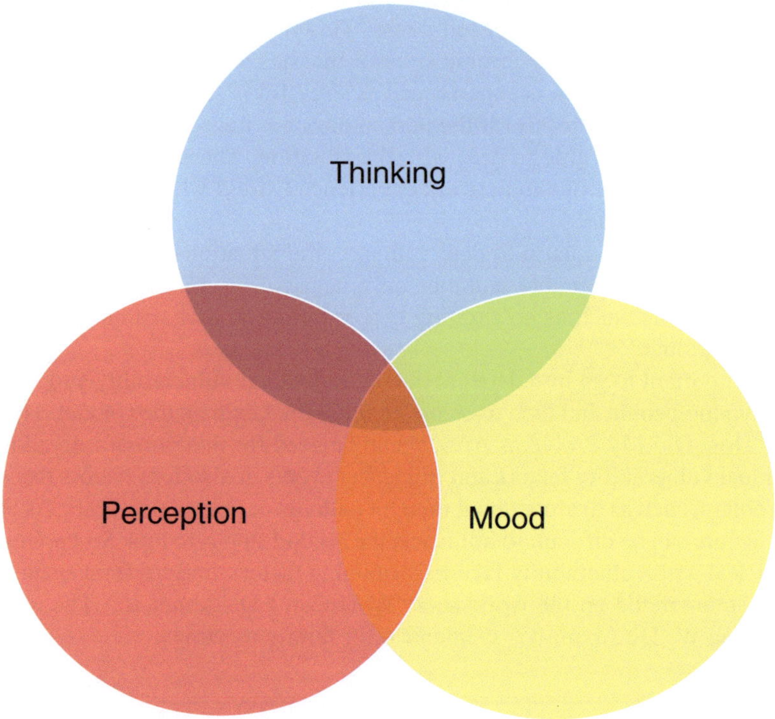

Fig. 4.1 Worksheet 1 to Worksheet 6

How Does Psychosis Develop?

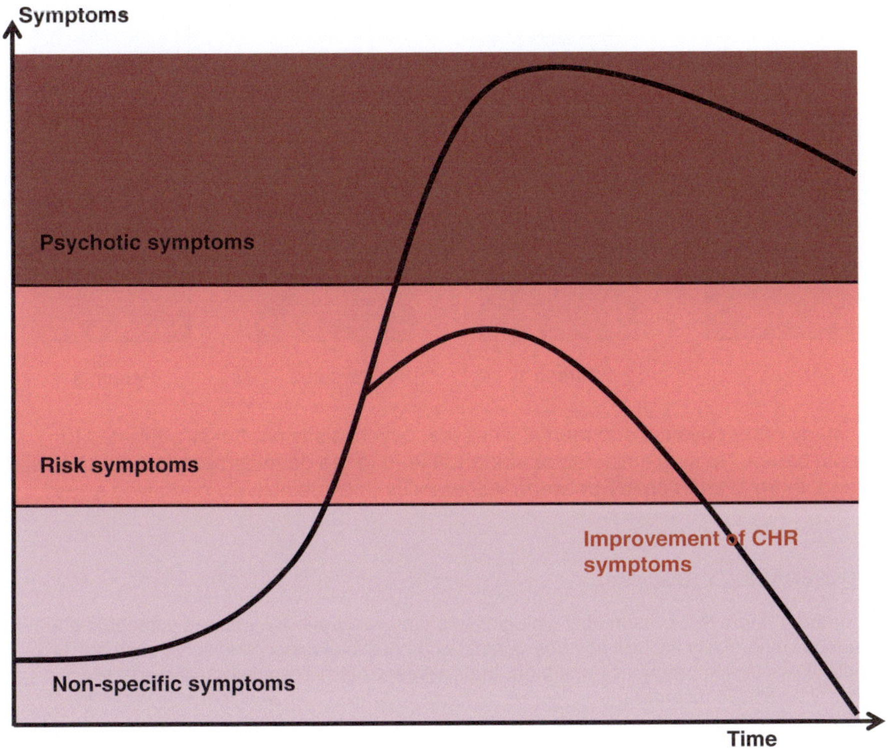

Fig. 4.1 (continued)

What Causes Psychosis?

The Stress-Vulnerability Model

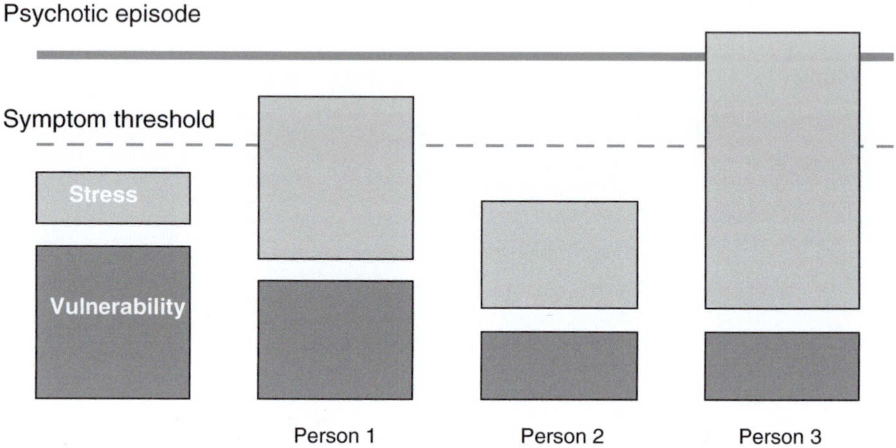

Like many other physical and mental illnesses, psychosis is not easily attributed to a single cause. No single risk factor alone will lead to the development of a psychosis. Instead, there is an interplay between vulnerability and subjectively perceived stress.

1. VULNERABILITY (Diathesis)

Vulnerability refers to a presumably biologically-based susceptibility. Factors contributing to increased vulnerability include adverse genetic and neurobiological conditions, such as complications during pregnancy and birth, brain diseases (e.g. meningitis), and a family history of psychotic disorders.

2. STRESS (Subjective Stress)

Stress refers to psychological and social demands that are experienced as highly stressful. Chronic excessive stress and, in particular, critical life events can trigger psychosis if there is a corresponding vulnerability.

Fig. 4.1 (continued)

How Did my Problems Start?

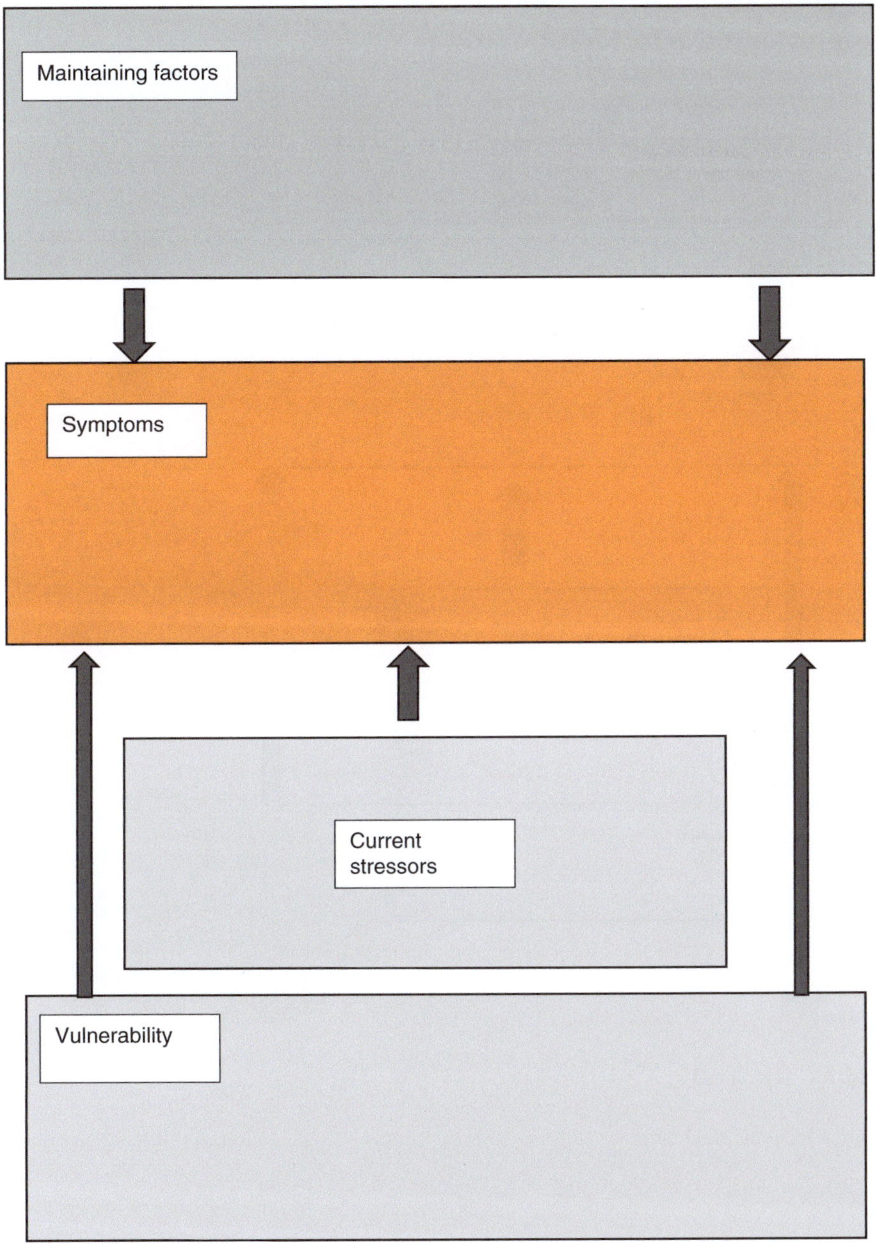

Fig. 4.1 (continued)

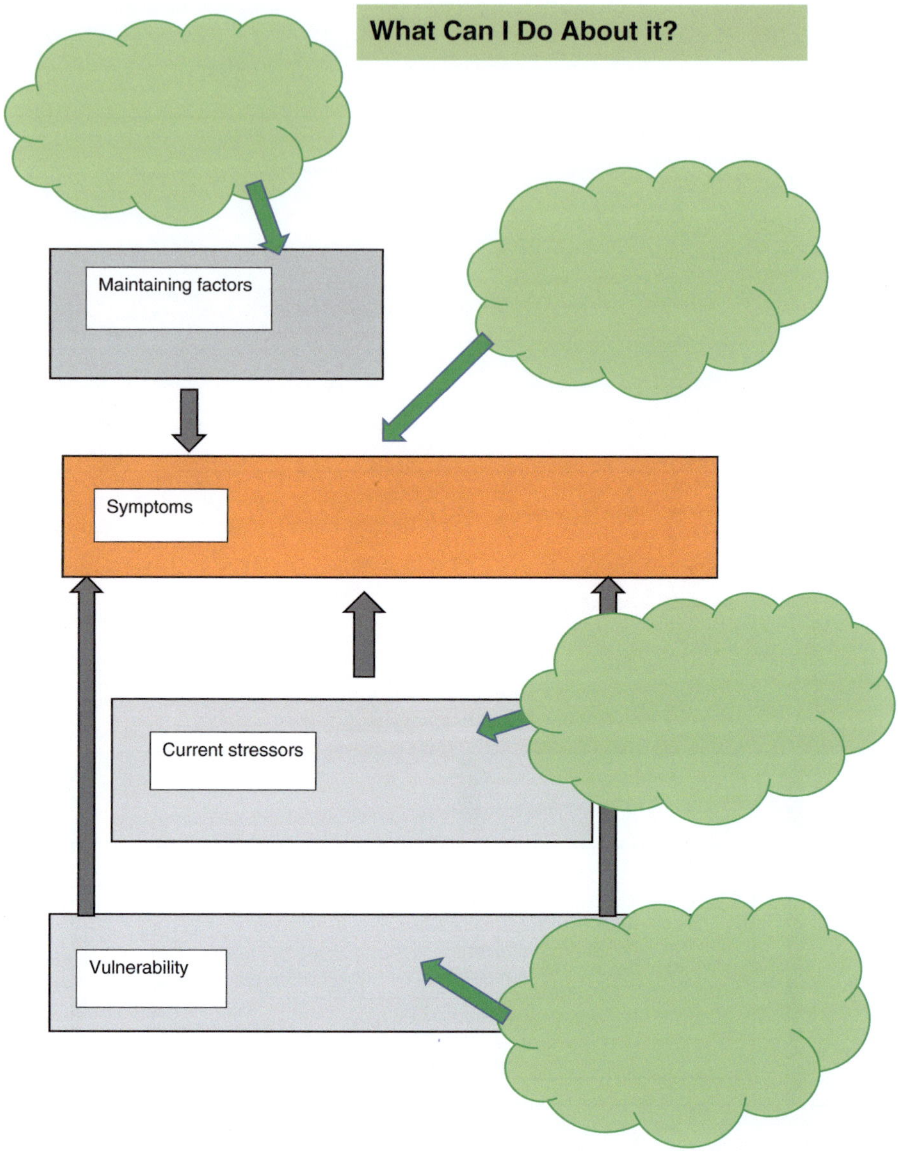

Fig. 4.1 (continued)

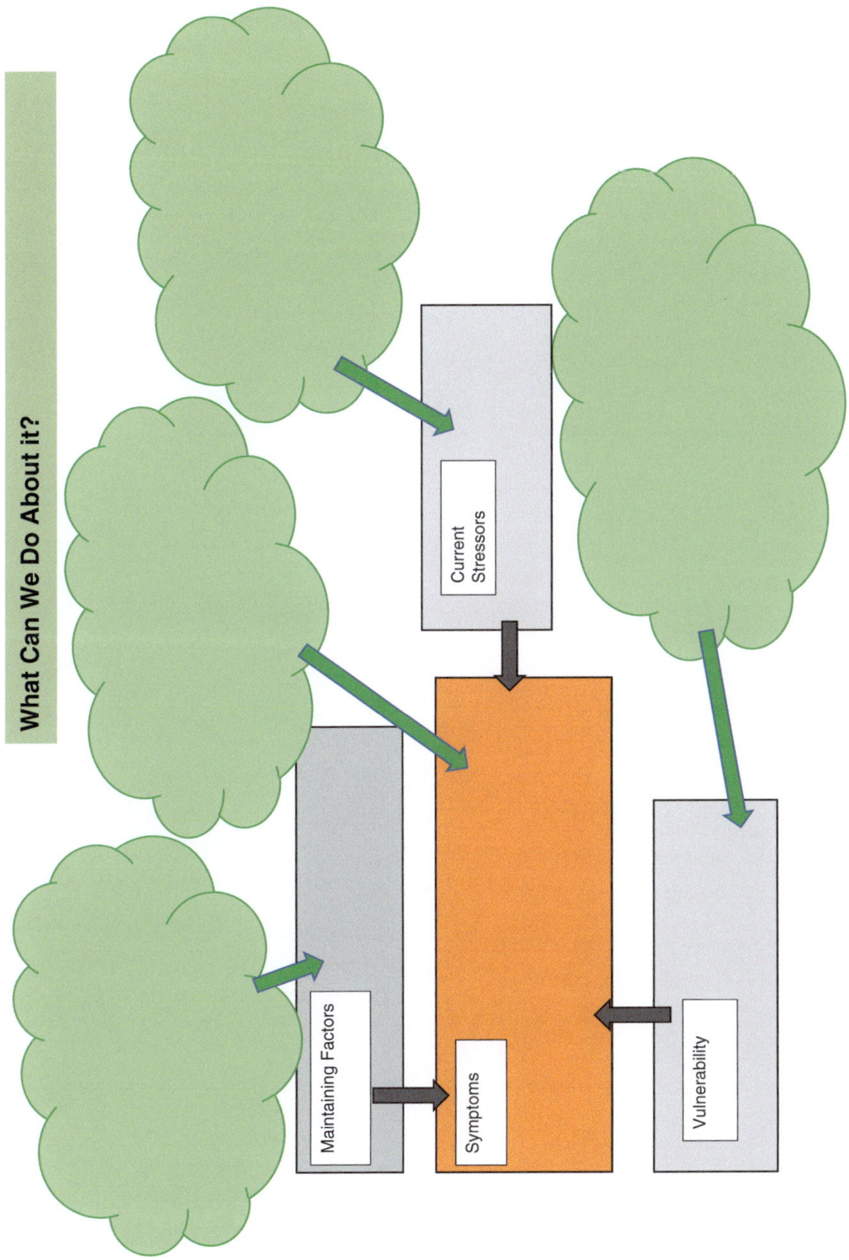

Fig. 4.1 (continued)

Symptom Management 5

5.1 General Information on Therapeutic Work with CHR Symptoms

Especially at the beginning of treatment, most patients feel insecure when dealing with the symptoms of CHR. In addition to feeling the considerable distress caused by the symptoms themselves, they often experience a strong fear of worsening symptoms. To avoid increasing uncertainty, the therapist should be careful not to react inappropriately (e.g., with disbelief, insecurity, irritation, or trivialization) to symptom reports, whether through body language, interruptions, or reassurances. These would only make the patient feel even more insecure.

It is also recommended to use the patient's own terms to describe the symptoms. For example, if the patient describes derealization as "perceptual disturbances," this term can be used. If the patient speaks of "voices," the therapist can also speak of "voices," but if the patient says "whispering," it would be better to use the word "whispering."

5.1.1 Better Understanding of the Symptoms

The foundations for a better understanding of symptoms are established during the diagnostic phase. During that stage, it is worth taking the time to identify risk symptoms and their occurrence patterns. It can also be helpful to create an individual explanatory model for the symptoms together with the patient (see worksheet "How Did My Problems Arise?"). Working alongside the patient allows the therapist to provide continuous feedback about the possible correlation between the symptoms

---

Supplementary Information The online version contains supplementary material available at https://doi.org/10.1007/978-3-032-10341-3_5. The videos can be accessed individually by clicking the DOI link in the accompanying figure caption or by scanning this link with the SN More Media App.

N. Traber-Walker, M. Franscini, *Adolescents at Clinical High Risk for Psychosis*,
https://doi.org/10.1007/978-3-032-10341-3_5

and certain life events (e.g., stress). Once CHR symptoms have been identified, it is important to emphasize that, while they require treatment, they can indeed be treated. Worksheets with brief psychoeducation are available on both the most important CHR symptoms and the most common comorbid symptoms, which can be discussed with patients during therapy sessions and given to them to take home.

- **Symptoms:** The section "symptoms" in the Robin Z app contains information and coping strategies for the different CHR symptoms and the most common comorbid symptoms. This allows patients to access the information at any time and read advice on symptom management when symptoms occur, empowering them to better cope with their symptoms.
- **Own coping strategies:** In addition to the predefined symptom management tips, patients can record their own coping strategies or supportive statements from therapy under 'Memo.'
- **Further symptoms:** In addition to the predefined symptoms, patients can define their own symptoms with a short psychoeducational text and coping strategies. The patient's own symptoms can also be recorded in the logbook.

Tutorial video "**Symptoms**" (Fig. 5.1) discusses the use of the function in the therapy session.

5.1.2 Acceptance of the Symptoms

Experience from early detection consultations shows that some symptoms can persist and do not improve even with prolonged treatment. In the case of such persistent symptoms, therapy aims to find a way of dealing with them that minimizes their impact on everyday life.

Most people with CHR symptoms are worried about becoming psychotic. To counter this fear, it can be useful to keep a log of symptoms and to define non-worsening as a good sign. Learning to categorize the symptom as "just a symptom with no impact on reality" can improve the patient's quality of life despite persistent symptoms. This may mean, for example, that a patient hears voices but recognizes them as unreal and can therefore ignore them to the extent that they have minimal impact on their daily life.

5.1.3 Restoring the Ability to Act

Patients should be taught how to better cope with their symptoms as quickly as possible so that the state of being helpless in the face of symptoms can be disrupted. The therapeutic challenge is to find a balance between the desire to get rid of the

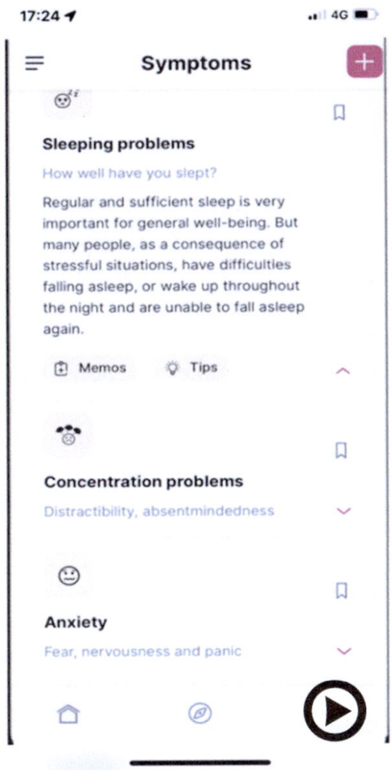

Fig. 5.1 Tutorial video "Symptoms" (▶ https://doi.org/10.1007/000-k5g)

symptoms and the acceptance of the symptoms. Adolescents suffering from CHR symptoms need to feel that they can take small steps to positively influence their symptoms.

During the sessions, the different strategies for managing and reducing symptoms are discussed. For these, the already mentioned worksheets on symptom management are useful. The aim is to discuss the application and purpose of the strategies with the patient during the treatment session. Patients are then encouraged to try some of the suggestions on the worksheets by next week. It is recommended to try several strategies, but not all at once. It is more effective if patients choose a few strategies and discuss their effectiveness at the next session.

A strategy that is perceived as ineffective if it does not produce immediate results can easily be discarded by the patient. This is why the individual strategies should be discussed before and after the session, as such an early or immediate discarding may not yet be appropriate.

The following questions are therefore helpful:

- Can you see how this advice might help?
- Have you ever tried it? Was it helpful?

- Why do you think it didn't work? How did you do it?
- Do you have any other strategies or tips that are not on the list?

5.2 Treatment of CHR Symptoms

CHR symptoms refer to changes in affect, drive, perception, and cognition that are reminiscent of early symptoms of psychosis. As only disturbances in perception and cognition are considered to be indicative of CHR for psychosis, symptoms in these two categories must be present to meet CHR criteria. CHR symptoms are similar to psychosis-specific symptoms such as delusions, disorganized thinking, or hallucinations, though in a milder form. Unlike psychotic patients, people with CHR symptoms are still able to recognize and challenge their symptoms as unreal. However, they can be very distressed by the symptoms and suffer greatly as a result.

Changes in affect and impulsivity alone are not sufficient for meeting CHR criteria, as they are not specific and can be seen in other disorders, such as depression. Nevertheless, the majority of people with CHR symptoms also show changes in drive or affect. It is often these symptoms that lead to consultation with a specialist since they have a significant impact on daily functioning and cause high levels of distress.

5.2.1 Alteration in Affect and Drive

It is often difficult to distinguish whether changes in drive and affect are part of CHR for psychosis (so-called adynamia or prodrome of negative symptoms) or a manifestation of a depressive episode. This is particularly the case as many patients with CHR symptoms also meet the criteria for depression. Additionally, the cognitive and perceptual disturbances can also lead to depressive symptoms, often causing feelings of despair, anxiety, or hopelessness. Whether mood changes are considered a CHR symptom or a comorbid depressive episode, the treatment approach is the same.

At this point, we will briefly discuss the changes in affect and drive that are often observed in early intervention centers. Typical symptoms in adolescents meeting CHR criteria include a blunted affect and anhedonia. Many patients describe a strong indifference to the point of being numb. It is also commonly reported that they feel less affection for their family and/or friends than they did previously. This can lead to intense distress and feelings of guilt.

An inability to distinguish between different emotions is also often reported. Unlike numbness, the patients experience a feeling but are unable to identify whether it is anger, fear, or sadness; all emotions feel the same. In some cases, they cannot even categorize whether they are experiencing a positive or unpleasant sensation.

Working on awareness of feelings is, therefore, an important part of therapy. Physical exercises and mindfulness exercises are suitable for this.

Many patients meeting CHR criteria report a marked lack of energy and drive, also known as adynamia. This is typically characterized by a general lack of energy, rapid exhaustion during daily activities, or an inability to engage in goal-directed activities. There is also often a general slowing down, which can affect thinking, movement (motor skills), or even speech. In some cases, this slowing cannot be observed externally but is only subjectively felt by the patient, as the activities mentioned above require more effort and strength than they previously did.

Due to symptoms, particularly in the areas of mood and drive, many patients experience limited functioning and show impairment in their daily school or work life. It is important to discuss with patients and their parents how their daily routine can be maintained. Allowing patients to take sick leave is only advisable in exceptional cases, as symptoms often worsen in the absence of daily structure. It is more beneficial to discuss with the patient and their family how to maintain a daily structure and how to meaningfully relieve their daily challenges. Goals and expectations should be adapted to the patient's current state of mind. For example, a goal may be for a patient to continue attending school, even if they are not currently able to meet performance expectations. It is worth contacting teachers or employers to discuss individual solutions, such as a temporary exemption from grades.

A first step in the treatment of mood swings is to show patients the connection between emotions, thoughts, and behavior (Fig. 5.2). Therefore, using specific everyday examples to explain the interactions between these three areas is helpful.

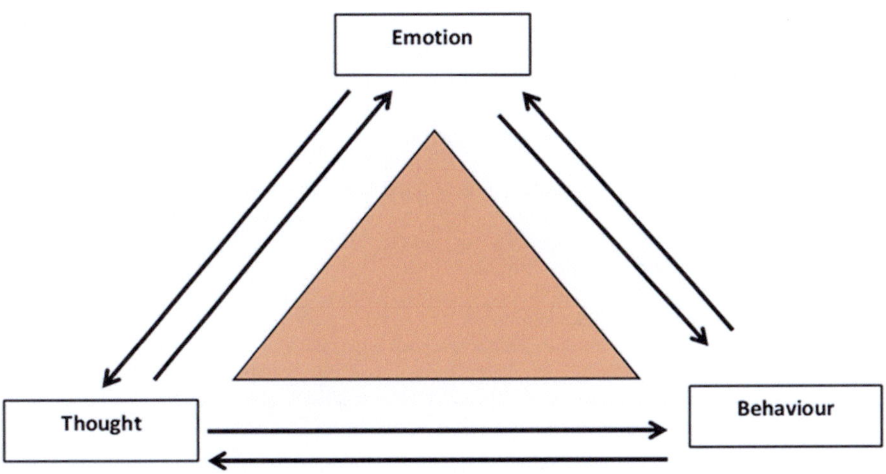

Fig. 5.2 Interconnection between thoughts–behavior–emotion

Therapeutic Conversation with Lucy

Lucy's calendar notes that she has dance class tonight. She hasn't been for a fortnight.

Thoughts:	I haven't gone twice already. I definitely can't do the choreography anymore, and everyone else will be so much better than I am.
***Emotion*:**	Lucy has been feeling bad all day anyway. She feels sad, unloved, and insecure. When she thinks about how she could embarrass herself while dancing, she feels like bursting into tears. She has an uneasy, sinking feeling in her stomach.
***Behavior*:**	Lucy decides to stay at home and not go to dance class. Consequently, the thought remains that she can't manage anything, and she feels like a real failure. Lucy feels even more worthless now.

The following week, Lucy comes to therapy and says that she is considering quitting dancing. She has missed three lessons. She does not think she'll be able to go this week. The therapist knows that dancing is actually very important to Lucy and that the hobby is very good for her. The therapist, therefore, tries to use this example to address the interplay between thoughts, emotions, and behavior.

The therapist's support of Lucy in questioning her thoughts about dancing could lead to the following perspective from Lucy: I haven't been to dance class three times now, so I'll probably be a bit worse at the choreography. I know that if I go there today, it will be really difficult in the beginning, but I've always been one of the better dancers in the group, so by the end of the class, I will have caught up with the others. I will have mastered the choreography. If I really try, it could be good.

How will Lucy feel when she goes to dance class and actually gets the choreography right by the end of the lesson? Exhausted and tired, probably, but that's how she feels every night, no matter what she's done. Only, instead of a sense of failure, there might be a sense of pride or joy.

Therapeutic Conversation with Lucy

Lucy:	I've missed so much—three lessons already. I can't keep up with it.
Therapist:	That's a shame. You used to be a very good dancer, weren't you?
Lucy:	Yes, I think so.
Therapist:	You think so? I remember your mum once said that your dance teacher described you as very talented.
Lucy:	Yes, that's true. I was actually one of the better dancers in the group, but now I've missed a lot and I certainly can't keep up with the choreography.
Therapist:	Do you learn the choreography very quickly?
Lucy:	*(nods)* I have no trouble with that.
Therapist:	Others in the course surely do.
Lucy:	*(smiles)* yes, some take longer.
Therapist:	Does it happen often that someone misses a class?
Lucy:	Yes, of course, that happens. That's not so bad. Many parts of the choreography are repeated, and we have time to practice. The teacher is also patient and is happy to show us everything again.
Therapist:	So it's not so bad if you miss a class.
Lucy:	No. but I missed three classes.
Therapist:	How do you think the class would go if you went today?
Lucy:	I wasn't there three times. I missed three parts of the choreography, which means it would be difficult.

Therapist:	You say it would be difficult. That doesn't mean it's *impossible*.
Lucy:	No, of course not. But it would be very exhausting. And I would have a lot of trouble at the beginning.
Therapist:	Do you think you could catch up with the others by the end of the lesson? I mean, dancing is easy for you.
Lucy:	By the end of the class, if I really make an effort, I probably will.
Therapist:	How would you feel if you were caught up by the end of the class?
Lucy:	Good, I think.
Therapist:	What feeling would you experience?
Lucy:	Pride, I think.
Therapist:	So you would be proud. How do you think you'll feel if you go home after your therapy session today and don't go to dance class?
Lucy:	Hm, not better. Probably bad.
Therapist:	What do you think would be the worst thing that could happen when you go to dance class?
Lucy:	That I don't know the choreography at the beginning.
Therapist:	Why would that be bad?
Lucy:	I don't know... Maybe it's not so bad.

5.2.1.1 Depressive Symptoms

The major challenge in addressing depressive symptoms in therapy is that patients often feel helpless in the face of these symptoms, making it difficult for them to accept therapeutic input.

It is essential to address the patient's individual needs without overwhelming them. Their negative problem focus should be interrupted in a supportive and non-directive way that maintains appreciation and respect.

For example, appropriate sentences in therapy could be:

- You really don't have it easy; that's obvious. At the same time, I wonder if...
- Yes, that sounds extremely difficult. However, could it be that...
- This situation seems annoying. You're probably right that there's not much you can do about it. It seems like there's nothing you can do besides accept it, which is really difficult, I know. Are there other parts in your life where you think you can have more influence?

The primary therapeutic goals for patients with depressive symptoms are to interrupt dysfunctional thoughts and to promote engagement in daily life. The tips provided in the depression worksheets focus primarily on these two areas.

Impact techniques are helpful when working with patients with depressive symptoms (see Beaulieu and Hoff 2013). Here, visual metaphors are used to activate several senses simultaneously, allowing therapy content to be better internalized. In the treatment of patients with depressive symptoms, visualization can be a very effective therapeutic tool. For example, images, such as the triangle shown above, can be used to explain certain processes. Additionally, noting down keywords mentioned by patients and then examining them together can also be helpful. A therapist who initiates a certain activity can also serve as a good model for activating behavior.

The first recommended step in addressing dysfunctional thoughts is to work with the patient to identify their core beliefs about themselves and the world. Negative core beliefs are considered to be one of the main triggers for depressive episodes and contribute to the persistence of symptoms. Therefore, they are an important component of the individual explanation model (see worksheet "How Did My Problems Arise?"). While many adult patients have already strongly internalized their negative core beliefs, these beliefs are often adaptable and less stable in adolescent patients. For this reason, attitudes should be revisited repeatedly throughout the course of therapy. Children often adopt the beliefs and attitudes of their caregivers without questioning them. During the process of detachment from caregivers during puberty, these attitudes are usually questioned for the first time, and the adolescents begin to form their own opinions and beliefs. Peers often play a significant role in this process, as adolescents' self-image is heavily shaped by how they believe they are perceived by others. Patients with depressive symptoms usually have a negative image of themselves and their social status. In the case of adolescents meeting CHR criteria, the interpretation of their CHR symptoms increases the negative effect on their self-image. They feel anxious about their symptoms, worry that they are losing control of themselves, and doubt their ability to trust their own thoughts (see also Sects. 5.2.2 "Perceptive Disturbances" and 5.2.3.1 "Cognitive Disturbances"). In most cases, individuals do not want those around them to become aware of their symptoms. One reason is the fear of being labeled as "crazy." Additionally, many adolescents with CHR symptoms are highly suspicious, concealing their symptoms due to uncertainty about whom they can still trust. These factors should be carefully considered when addressing depressive cognition. It is therefore important to ask patients how they perceive their CHR symptoms and how this perception affects their self-image. Depending on how the patient responds to such questions, the focus in therapy may be less on typical depressive cognitions and more on paranoid thoughts. More details on how to deal with dysfunctional thoughts are described in Chap. 6.

Encouraging patients to be more active in everyday life despite depression is a therapeutic challenge that requires a great deal of sensitivity. Patients need to be challenged, but they should not be overwhelmed. Excessive demands often lead to even greater exhaustion. Underchallenging, however, can have the same effect. As described at the beginning of the chapter, the structure of daily life should be adapted to the current state of mind. Patients require a daily structure to facilitate any potential improvement in mood. To-do lists and daily plans are helpful in achieving these goals, as they help both with structuring and the feeling of achievement associated with accomplishment. The worksheet "Weekly Goals" is suitable for working with patients with depressive symptoms. It helps individuals to act and conveys a sense of achievement. More on the topic of everyday structure is described in Chap. 7, "Everyday Activation." The concept of "sense of achievement" is crucial. Patients with depressive symptoms often tend to set overly ambitious and unrealistic goals themselves. This regularly leads to feelings of defeat and failure because they do not fulfill their own expectations. In therapy, these high expectations should be actively scrutinized by the therapist. Instead of overly ambitious goals, realistic daily plans should be made.

It is also important to work with patients on accepting their current reduced performance abilities. Comparisons with somatic illnesses can be helpful here. Nobody would think of running a marathon with a broken leg. It is just as impossible to perform at your best in everyday life when suffering from acute depression. Maintaining a school or work routine despite depression is a significant challenge that should be adequately acknowledged.

Therapeutic Conversation with Lucy

Lucy:	I didn't do any work for school last night. I didn't study anything, even though we have two exams at the end of this week.
Therapist:	What did you do instead?
Lucy:	Nothing. I was way too exhausted. I watched three episodes of a new series on Netflix. I should have been studying.
Therapist:	And then? Did you go to sleep?
Lucy:	No, at some point, my mom came into the room and asked me if I wanted another cup of tea. Then I went into the living room and drank tea with her and my sister.
Therapist:	And was that nice?
Lucy:	It was fun. All three of us were tired and joked around a bit. I was even able to sleep really well afterwards.
Therapist:	And how were you feeling this morning?
Lucy:	A little better. I felt less exhausted and had more energy, but as soon as I got to school, my mood took a turn for the worse. I remembered that we have two exams at the end of the week and that I should have studied yesterday.
Therapist:	Listening to you, I get the impression that last night was actually good for you and was exactly what you needed.
Lucy:	Well, yes. But I really should have studied.
Therapist:	Lucy, let's say a friend told you that she couldn't study yesterday because she had the flu. Today she still feels exhausted and weak, but she has some exams this week. What advice would you give her?
Lucy:	I would tell her to get some rest and go to bed early because she's not feeling well. There's no point in studying when she won't be productive anyway. She should get some rest and study tomorrow when she's feeling a little bit better.
Therapist:	But you're not doing well at the moment either. Why are you being so hard on yourself?
Lucy:	That's different. She really is ill.
Therapist:	You too; that's why you come to me for therapy. Why is there such a big difference? You're just as limited in your ability to perform at the moment, albeit for different reasons. Yesterday evening seems to have done you good, and right now, it's very important that you recover. Just as you wouldn't expect your friend with the flu to be able to study, you shouldn't expect yourself to be able to. Just like her, you need to recover. And you might even manage to study better tonight because you didn't do anything yesterday.
Lucy:	It's just that I always had good grades and prepared a lot for exams.
Therapist:	How are your grades at the moment?
Lucy:	Not so good anymore.
Therapist:	But good enough?
Lucy:	Well, mostly yes.
Therapist:	Even though you are learning less than before? Because you are less able to concentrate?
Lucy:	Yes.
Therapist:	I know that's difficult to accept, and you'd like to continue being such a good student. But even though you're not doing perfectly right now, you're still getting good enough grades. In my eyes, that's a huge achievement that you should be proud of.
Lucy:	Yes. I didn't think about it that way. I guess you're right.

5.2.1.2 (Hypo-)manic Symptoms

Severe mood swings are very common in patients with CHR symptoms. Overall, patients with (hypo-)manic symptoms are at an increased risk of developing psychosis. (Hypo-)manic symptoms must therefore be monitored carefully.

(Hypo-)manic symptoms can also be precursors to a psychotic episode. The transition between manic and psychotic ideations of grandeur can be seen as a continuum. An important distinguishing feature is that although manic ideations of grandeur involve an overestimation of one's own abilities, they are usually still coherent in themselves and not entirely fabricated or imagined. Psychotic ideas of grandeur often contain illogical thought processes or even magical, impossible components. A teenager with mania who can sing well might describe themselves as one of the best singers ever, perhaps even chosen by God to make the world happy through song. On the other hand, a teenager with psychosis and a talent for singing might be convinced that they are destined to bring peace between Israel and Palestine through music. They may attribute the quality of their voice not to the fact of numerous completed singing lessons but to a large, white dove of peace that appeared to them one evening and granted them a good voice.

It can also be difficult to distinguish between (hypo-)manic symptoms and age-appropriate adolescent euphoria. In fact, the teenage years are characterized by strong mood swings, and overconfidence and risky behavior are not uncommon in adolescence. The diagnosis of a (hypo-)manic episode should not be given lightly. In contrast to adolescents with normal pubertal mood swings, patients with mania are almost impossible to reach emotionally, and any objections from their caregivers are typically ignored.

The first step in therapy is to identify a list of warning signs by which the young person can recognize that their mood is threatening to tip over into a high. These can be very small changes, such as a sudden reduced awareness of basic needs, an increased urge to move, or a tendency to speak and think faster. Since it is often challenging for patients to recognize changes early on, input from caregivers can be especially helpful in identifying warning signs.

Patients with a tendency towards (hypo-)manic symptoms are advised to avoid stimulating substances such as caffeine, illegal drugs, and alcohol as much as possible. It is useful to discuss with patients how they organize their evenings and recover from everyday life. Regular sleep and rest are important; bedtime rituals and sleep protocols can be very helpful to achieve this. A reduced need for sleep is often the first warning sign of an impending new mood high. Additionally, relaxation and mindfulness exercises (see Chap. 8)—if used regularly—can prevent highs or help patients calm down at the first signs of mood swings.

In general, patients who are prone to (hypo-)manic symptoms are advised not to take on too much. Such guidance from a therapist may give patients the impression that the therapist is trying to slow them down, to which they can react angrily. A detailed psychoeducation explaining why it is necessary for them to exercise restraint is therefore essential. With hypomanic symptoms in particular, patients often experience little or no distress. However, (hypo-)manic moods often lead to problematic behaviors, such as frequent socializing, substance use, unprotected sexual activity, and opposition to authority figures like teachers or employers. These behaviors negatively impact the patient's daily life, add stress, and ultimately exacerbate CHR symptoms.

Therapeutic Conversation with Michael

Therapist:	What are the first signs you notice that indicate that your mood is changing and another high is imminent?
Michael:	I suddenly feel more hyperactive. I can hardly sit still and have a strong urge to move.
Therapist:	Are those some of the first signs?
Michael:	Yes, I think so. And that I feel more self-confident and popular. I really enjoy being around people and find it hard to be alone.
Therapist:	Are there any other signs?
Michael:	Well, my sleep is affected during both the low moods and the high moods. And I feel more irritable. I'm more argumentative during the highs and have a tendency to get easily offended.
Therapist:	Is there any way you can stop the highs?
Michael:	During the highs, I tend to take on a lot of things at once and am overactive. But in reality, it would probably be good if I withdrew a little and got a little peace and quiet.
Therapist:	Have you ever tried this?
Michael:	The problem is that I can't think as clearly when I'm experiencing a high. And it's difficult to be alone then, which is why I go out a lot.
Therapist:	I understand that it's difficult to withdraw when you're experiencing a high. I think you need to act beforehand when you start to notice the first signs and when you feel more hyperactive. Instead of acting on this impulse, do something quiet and rest.

5.2.1.3 Irritability

Many adolescents meeting CHR criteria experience extreme irritability and describe a strong sense of suffering as a result. They can suddenly become intensely angry over trivial matters. Increased irritability is a nonspecific risk symptom for psychosis. This means that increased irritability often occurs in the prodrome, but it is too nonspecific to be considered a clear risk symptom for psychosis, as it is common in a number of disorders. In children and adolescents in particular, irritability is also a symptom of a depressive episode.

Mood swings from being content and balanced to angry and aggressive are a normal part of adolescence. Even teenagers who were seen by their parents as easy-going and emotionally stable during childhood can become highly irritable and react impulsively to minor issues during their teenage years. Subsequently, it is very difficult to distinguish between normal pubertal phenomena and pathological irritability. A mood diary or recording the context and occurrence of irritable episodes can provide important information on baseline irritability levels. In treatment, it is important to assess whether irritability consistently occurs alongside other symptoms. This concept will be illustrated with two common CHR symptoms:

- **Hearing voices**
  Patients meeting CHR criteria are often much more irritable during phases in which they hear voices. There can be various reasons for this:
  - Simply processing auditory hallucinations heightens general sensitivity. Imagine dealing with an added layer of noise, like a constant murmur of voices or even shouting in daily life—it quickly becomes clear how much it would reduce one's tolerance. If you haven't experienced this, try spending an hour with a poorly tuned radio station in the background (static and overlapping voices) to get a sense of the discomfort.
  - Fighting the hallucinations also requires a lot of energy. Inner disputes with the voices can overlap with actual disputes with another person.
  - The voices can turn patients against those around them. Statements like, "See, I told you your friends are all against you," amplify the patient's anger even further in that moment.
- **Distrust**
  Increased irritability can also be caused by distrust or even paranoid thoughts. Due to a tendency to self-reference, patients with CHR symptoms can feel judged or threatened by their environment, even if there is no real reason for such assumptions. The techniques of hypothetical reasoning (see Chap. 6) can help in dealing with "paranoid" irritability.

Regardless of the cause of the increased irritability, it can lead to impulsive outbursts, which can have negative consequences. Therefore, it is important to identify the recognizable warning signs that lead to impulsive outbursts during therapy.

The therapist should address this issue openly with the patient and suggest strategies for dealing with irritability and impulsive outbursts. Breathing exercises, muscle tension and relaxation, or the use of an anger ball, for example, are helpful.

Therapeutic Conversation with Michael

Michael:	I've been having outbursts of anger very often recently. They are usually completely inappropriate. I blow up over little things. The other day, I got so angry at the checkout in the supermarket just because a woman pushed in front of me. I shouted at the woman, and everyone around me looked at me in horror. I was so ashamed.
Therapist:	Are these outbursts of anger completely new to you?
Michael:	Well, I was like that as a younger child, too—Impulsive. I got angry quickly, was always arguing with everyone, and often said or did things that I regretted afterwards. As I got older, I was able to control myself better.
Therapist:	How did you manage that back then?
Michael:	It's a bit unpleasant, but I remember my bench neighbor in elementary school telling me, "you're always so aggressive. If the rest of us have an argument or we don't like something, we talk about it. But you always use your fists straight away." that stuck with me, and from that day on, I made a firm resolution not to react so impulsively again.
Therapist:	But you still had the rage impulses?
Michael:	Yes, I clenched my fists as tightly as I could in those situations. I imagined how I would lash out at the other person and hit them with my fists. Then I let go and felt better again.

Therapist:	That trick with the clenched fists—Do you still do that today?
Michael:	Not really. At some point, it worked without the fists. At some point, I even managed to stop imagining how I would hit the other person.
Therapist:	Really? No such images of revenge in your head?
Michael:	Well, not quite. Sometimes I imagined myself breaking something that belonged to the person. Or how I would verbally embarrass them in front of others. But I never really said anything because I knew that my verbal reaction would be too extreme at that moment.
Therapist:	I really like your trick with the fist. However, you should release the tension as soon as possible. You can always repeat the clenching and releasing as many times as needed. By tensing your fist and then releasing it, your body relaxes again. You follow the physical impulse of anger, which satisfies that desire. By letting go, your body also relaxes again. Try it out.
Michael:	*(tightens his fist and lets go; he does this exercise three times)*
Therapist:	And do you notice a difference?
Michael:	Yes, a little bit. But I don't know if it would be good to tense my fists in an angry situation. What if I go off on someone?
Therapist:	That's why letting go is an important part of the exercise. But if that feels too unsafe for you, you can also tense your toes to achieve a similar effect. Or you can even tense all the muscles in your body. I call it the spaghetti method, or spaghetti body, because you tense your whole body as much as spaghetti in a packet.

To reduce irritability overall, it is important to lead as healthy a lifestyle as possible with sufficient sleep, regular meals, and exercise. At the same time, however, the therapist should normalize the experience of irritability. Everyone is familiar with moments when they can tolerate less. Especially in particular chaotic instances, it is normal to feel more irritable.

The feeling of anger or annoyance does not have to be seen as negative per se. Pronounced feelings of anger occur, above all, when a lot of frustration has built up. It is worth discussing in therapy what might be behind the anger. There is often an understandable reason for increased irritability that needs to be taken seriously. If patients always ignore their actual needs and only combat irritability superficially, the irritability cannot decrease at all.

5.2.2 Perceptive Disturbances

Patients who suffer from perceptual disturbances usually describe a very high level of distress because these symptoms are particularly worrying and very unsettling. This makes it even more important to explain to patients that changes in perception do not necessarily mean that they are suffering from a psychotic disorder. Symptoms such as hearing voices can also occur temporarily in the general population and are not at all uncommon, especially in adolescence.

5.2.2.1 Perceptual Abnormalities and Hallucinations

The most frequently reported perceptual symptom is hearing voices. Overall, auditory hallucinations are more common than visual hallucinations, but adolescents meeting CHR criteria often report a variety of visual perceptual changes, such as the perceived movement of stationary objects, photopsia, or metamorphopsia. Although these do not fulfill the quality of an optical hallucination, they are experienced as distressing.

The following aspects are important in the treatment of hallucinations:

- Detailed psychoeducation.
- Changing metacognitive beliefs about the hallucinations.
- Coping strategies for dealing with hallucinations.
- Interventions to reduce enduring conditions, such as stress.

In a first step, individual factors that contribute to the development of perceptive disturbances should be assessed:

- When did the changes in perception first occur?
- In which situations do they occur?
- At what times of day do they occur?
- How long do they normally last?
- Are the perceptive disturbances also experienced in the presence of other people or only when the patient is alone?

In order for the therapist to gain a more accurate impression of the symptoms, it is recommended that symptom logs be completed. In addition to the frequency and intensity of the symptoms, situational factors and associated feelings, thoughts, and coping strategies should be recorded. Symptom logs can make systematic patterns visible for the patient, e.g., changes in perception always occur in social situations, during the exam period, or when the family argues.

Another question arising when children and adolescents report perceptive disturbances may be: What could the symptoms be helpful for? Could the symptoms result in a hidden or secondary gain for the patient? The symptoms may represent a subconscious solution strategy. Hearing voices may provide an excuse or justification for certain actions. Younger patients may say that the voices ordered them to do something they actually wanted to do, such as hit their sibling or not tidy up their room. Patients who feel under pressure to perform at school may refer to voices as a reason why they are not able to perform well. The hallucinations may be to blame for the fact that they can no longer concentrate or learn.

Dysfunctional Beliefs

The adolescents' own theories and explanatory models regarding their changes in perception are of great importance for the treatment of symptoms. For example, voices that are interpreted as coming from the devil are much more threatening than those that are perceived by the patient as a malfunction of the brain. In addition to the patients themselves, family members must also be asked about their explanatory models, as the views of caregivers have a strong impact on the patient's experience.

Biological explanations for hallucinations often provide relief. The symptoms are perceived as less frightening. However, other patients are skeptical of biological explanations and stick to their own explanatory models. Delusional beliefs about perceptual changes can be challenged by hypothetical reasoning in the same way as delusional ideas. Other anxious worries without delusional components, such as "I'm going crazy. I'm losing control," should be taken seriously and acknowledged by the therapist while also being contextualized through a depathologizing approach.

Reality Testing

It is important to work with patients on as many reality testing strategies as possible. This may include:

- An understanding that the hallucinations are not real. They are temporary, false activations in certain areas of the brain.
- A pursuit of the perception: e.g., patients attempt to touch an optical hallucination. For illusions in the dark, they turn on the light. If the patient hears voices, they might stand against the wall in order to ask the question: Where could the voice be coming from if I am absolutely sure that nobody is standing behind me?
- Asking other people: If there really is a voice, shouldn't others be able to hear it too?
- A change of perspective for a moment: Plugging the ears to stop listening or closing the eyes to stop seeing. Are the hallucinations still there?
- Distinguishing the details: What distinguishes hallucinations from real perceptions? What do real voices sound like compared to "imaginary voices"? What about visual hallucinations? For example, many people report that, in visual hallucinations, the colors are paler or the image is more blurred. Other people may be able to identify a hallucination by details that are out of context. For example, the people in the hallucination may not be wearing shoes, or they may be wearing a cardigan when it is snowing, but they are not cold.
- Grounding exercises: Hallucinations can lead to dissociative states. Exercises to anchor the patient in the here and now can be helpful. Touching a wall or a tabletop is often enough to regain contact with reality.

Therapeutic Conversation with Michael

Michael:	It was bad yesterday evening. The voices were there for a very long time, and they were so loud. I almost couldn't stand it.
Therapist:	How did you endure it?
Michael:	I listened to music with headphones and turned the music up really loud.
Therapist:	Does listening to music always help?
Michael:	Most of the time. I concentrate on the music, and, at some point, the voices stop.
Therapist:	That sounds exhausting. I think it's impressive how well you deal with it.
Michael:	It's not easy. And yesterday it took quite a long time for the voices to finally stop. Sometimes I'm very afraid that one day I won't realize that the voices are just my imagination.
Therapist:	But, at the moment, you always know, right?
Michael:	Yes, so far I've been able to tell. If I get unsure, I lean against a wall so that I'm sure no one can be behind me and that I'm just imagining the voices.
Therapist:	I think that's a very good strategy on your part. How did you come up with that idea?
Michael:	*(shrugs)* I don't know. At some point, when it was particularly bad, I leaned against the wall and realized that it helped.

5.2.2.2 Derealization and Depersonalization

In derealization, the environment is experienced as alien and unreal; in depersonalization, it is the patient's own person that feels unknown.

Sample text on derealization/depersonalization written by a patient (Leo, name changed by the authors):

Who am I? I think you should first know how I feel, because in my opinion, emotions make the person. So the question is rather: How do you feel? I feel like a leaf in autumn that has been torn away from its "family tree" by the strong wind and is randomly fluttering through life. I no longer feel like myself. How do you feel when you suffer from depression and also lose reality in a gradual process, like sand through your hand?

I am not happy. I am not angry. I am not sad. I am not scared. What is a living being without emotions? Nothing. I am nothing. I am drifting in the direction of the water without a soul, while my soul has said goodbye to me and is swimming upstream. I have lost myself. I have lost Leo. All that remains is a lifeless shell. What remains is the new Leo. I take up the question "Who am I?" again and say: I don't know who is living inside me now. How could I? It's a new person. I have been reset to the level of a baby. I have to rediscover and get to know my body. I have to get to know myself again.

Patients with pronounced derealization and depersonalization symptoms often present to early intervention centers for psychosis. However, neither derealization nor depersonalization is specific to psychosis. Although many patients with psychosis experience derealization or depersonalization, both conditions can be comorbid with various disorders such as depression, anxiety, or post-traumatic stress disorder. At the same time, they are considered separate diagnoses according to ICD-10. Many young people report that they experienced such symptoms for the first time after cannabis use. In some cases, the symptoms do not go away for years and even get worse. This is why patients must be informed about cannabis as a possible trigger during the initial consultation and are encouraged to stop using it.

Depersonalization and derealization are an "as if" feeling: "As if I am no longer myself. As if the environment has changed. As if the people around me are strangers." The patient's awareness of reality is intact; it is only the sense of reality that has changed. The states of derealization and depersonalization are not visible from the outside; even the closest relatives sometimes do not notice these changes. It is important to distinguish that although patients fear losing control over themselves, they still have it and have never lost it.

With regard to the fear of developing psychosis, it can be helpful to look at the ICD-10 categories with the patient. Most psychotic clinical pictures are categorized under F2 or even F3 (depression with psychotic symptoms). Psychotic conditions are also described under F0 (organic disorders) and F1 (substance abuse). However, derealization and depersonalization syndromes are classified under F4. With the help of these categories, patients can be shown in a simple, factual way that the syndrome has more in common with anxiety and stress disorders than with psychosis. This fact is already reassuring for many patients.

Derealization and depersonalization are symptoms that are very resistant to treatment. Little is known about the symptoms, and there is sparse literature on them. Some patients only experience the symptoms for transient moments, while others report constant states of derealization and depersonalization. It is important to work with patients to accept these conditions and support them to live a normal life despite the symptoms.

A healthy lifestyle is helpful against the symptoms: no substance use, regular meals, enough sleep, regular daily structures, exercise, and avoiding stress. At the same time, it is important to ask patients about their needs. Thus, the therapist can work with them to find ways to live as healthy a life as possible without giving up too many experiences typical of their age. Of course, it would be great if they had regular bedtimes, but going out with friends and coming home late are also part of adolescence. Normal social behavior needs to be encouraged; many patients react to the symptoms with massive social withdrawal.

The worksheets contain a list of coping strategies. Most of the strategies are designed to distract from the situation or to augment the mood and train the conscious perception.

Physical activity can be very helpful, especially sports that require a high level of concentration and use several parts of the body, such as climbing. Many patients with severe depersonalization report having moments of clarity again when climbing, as they are challenged both mentally and physically.

Caution is advised with relaxation exercises. Meditative exercises carry the danger of intensifying the sense of derealization or depersonalization. In contrast, mindfulness exercises such as mindful walking or mindful activity can be helpful.

Therapeutic Conversation with Lucy

Lucy describes her derealization and depersonalization as "perceptual states." That is why the therapist also uses this word. It makes sense to use the terms that the patients define for their symptoms. At the same time, the official technical term is mentioned again at the beginning of the conversation to remind Lucy that her symptoms have a name and are already known as such in medicine.

Lucy:	In the last few weeks, I have increasingly experienced these perceptual states again.
Therapist:	By states of perception, do you mean derealization and depersonalization?
Lucy:	Yes, the depersonalizations in particular have become stronger recently. I'm afraid that I'm slowly losing control of myself and might do something bad. Everything I do feels fake and weird. When I look at myself in the mirror, it's as if I'm not that person. I almost can't stand it.
Therapist:	And what do you do then?
Lucy:	I try not to look in the mirror at times because it worries me too much.
Therapist:	Let me see if I'm understanding. It's like you're not that person, but you always know it's you?
Lucy:	Yes, of course, I know it's me. I can see myself in the mirror. It just feels so strange, and I can hardly stand the feeling. I'm scared that one day I won't recognize myself in the mirror anymore.
Therapist:	Has this ever happened before?
Lucy:	No.
Therapist:	And you've never lost control of yourself?
Lucy:	No.
Therapist:	Have you ever done something that you didn't want to do? Something against your will? In these states of perception?
Lucy:	No, never before.

Therapist:	How long have you experienced this? For a long time, right?
Lucy:	Yes, over a year now.
Therapist:	Has the feeling of no longer being yourself ever gotten stronger during this course of the year?
Lucy:	Yes, sometimes it's extremely strong, sometimes a little less so. And fortunately, the conditions are not always there.
Therapist:	The perceptual states suddenly disappear?
Lucy:	*(nods)* yes, suddenly they're gone. Just like they suddenly appear. I can't control it.
Therapist:	I know that enduring these perceptual states is extremely exhausting and difficult. I can see how unpleasant these states are for you, and I also think you are working extremely hard by continuing to function so well in everyday life despite these states. But I have not heard that you have ever lost control or that you have ever not known what is real and what is not. Is there any evidence from your experience that this can happen?
Lucy:	No, not yet. But what if one day I can no longer do that? When I no longer know what is real and what is not?
Therapist:	We both don't know if that will happen. I can't tell you that it won't happen either. Because we don't know. But at the moment, we both have no reason to assume that you will actually lose control of yourself. You've been experiencing these conditions for over a year now. They occur frequently and have become more intense during this time. And yet, it has never happened that you have lost control of yourself. On the contrary, you have always known exactly what reality is and what is just a feeling.
Lucy:	(*agrees*) I'm so scared that I'm going to lose control of myself.
Therapist:	So it's mainly the fear of losing control? You have no indication that this could really happen, but it's actually a fear of it?
Lucy:	Yes, but it's very strong.
Therapist:	I believe you. And fear is a very, very unpleasant feeling. But fear is just a feeling. It's not reality, and it can't predict the future. Just because we are afraid that something will happen doesn't mean that it actually will. Many people were afraid that the world would end in 2000. And what happened on 1 January 2000?
Lucy:	*(smiles)* nothing at all.
Therapist:	Exactly. If we now look at your depersonalization states, we know they come and go. Enduring them is very, very unpleasant for you. But they are only temporary states, and they will pass. They don't hurt you; so far, there is no evidence that anything bad is happening to you because of these states. Perhaps in therapy, we can focus more on how you can endure these states? Preventing these states seems difficult. But we don't have to assume that they will get worse, and so far, there is no reason to believe that you will ever lose control of yourself.
Lucy:	*(nods)* yes, I think that's good.
Therapist:	You've been living with it for so long now; how have you managed to deal with these difficult conditions so far? What has helped you to endure them?
Lucy:	Hm. that varies. Distraction works. It helps when I write to friends or talk to my family. Although it takes a lot of effort for me at times to get in touch with others. I would prefer to retreat to my room and hide under the duvet.
Therapist:	Have you tried that?
Lucy:	Yes, of course. I hid, especially at the beginning. But that only made it worse. The fear of going crazy increased and became even stronger.
Therapist:	So, does it help you to socialize at times like this, even if it is difficult to do at first?
Lucy:	Yes, because it distracts me.

5.2.3 Changes in Cognition

CHR symptoms tend to occur during a period of challenging social development and vocational orientation. Losses in cognition can hinder the successful accomplishment of these developmental tasks, making it even more vital to address these symptoms.

The ability to think and learn is often impaired over a long period of time in the context of psychotic illness. This applies both to the period before an episode and the onset of the first psychotic symptoms, i.e., when risk symptoms occur, and the period after the episode. All areas of life can be affected, including everyday life at home, school, play, and leisure. This, of course, includes relationships and socializing with peers. Although people with CHR for psychosis do not reach the full diagnostic criteria, they often already suffer considerable cognitive and functional impairment.

The long-lasting but temporary changes lead to measurable performance losses in various intelligence and performance tests (IQ tests, concentration tests, etc.) with effects on everyday performance in school and vocational training. They contribute significantly to subjectively experienced distress and are even more important than the positive and negative symptoms that fluctuate over the course of the illness. As a result of the reduced absorption capacity, there is also less benefit from possible psycho- and socio-therapeutic offers (e.g., social skills training, behavioral therapy, or motivational groups).

According to current studies, the following areas are particularly affected: processing speed, attention, learning and memory, flexible thinking, planning, and action control.

The results of a meta-analysis by Fusar-Poli et al. (2012) show widespread cognitive impairments in people with an increased risk of psychosis compared to healthy individuals. These are visible in general intelligence, executive functions, verbal and visual memory, verbal fluency, attention, and working memory. Losses in the areas of verbal fluency and memory were most clearly associated with a psychotic crisis.

The impairment of basic cognitive abilities is the result of both the altered stimulus processing and the disturbed thinking and memory processes. In intelligence tests, the areas of fluid intelligence and declarative memory are particularly affected.

The connection between cognitive functions and psychosocial functioning is well documented, with significant effects on academic and occupational performance (see Green et al. 2004). Here, they are of greater significance than the positive and negative symptoms, which fluctuate in their severity over the course of the illness. However, the symptoms are often neglected in psychotherapy.

Treating these symptoms is very important, as they can lead to severe losses in academic or occupational performance and can also be a predictor of transitions to psychosis. One therapy method that addresses the area of "thinking" in detail is cognitive remediation (see also Chap. 7), which has become increasingly important in the treatment of psychotic patients over the last twenty years and has already been well evaluated.

Cognitive remediation is a form of behavioral training designed to improve cognitive processes (attention, memory, executive functions, and social cognition) sustainably and comprehensively through regular and intensive practice. The focus is on learning and thinking strategies. The statement "Bring the Brain to the Gym" can be used to compare cognitive remediation with muscle or skill-oriented training programs from the sports or fitness sector.

Positive effects are now documented, and cognitive remediation is recommended by medical associations. This is particularly true when cognitive training forms are combined with exercises for everyday life. New computer-based programs (e.g., virtual reality games) in this area are considered promising. However, there is a need for studies in this area.

Common elements of the various programs in this area are repeated practice, feedback on success, and a level of difficulty adapted to the current level of performance. Application in everyday situations is central to securing the learning progress achieved. For this reason, practice should also take place outside of therapy sessions. Assistance that is initially necessary is gradually reduced.

5.2.3.1 Cognitive Disturbances

The most frequently reported changes in formal thinking are:

- Slower thinking
- Blocked or racing thoughts
- Memory difficulties
- Concentration difficulties
- Receptive or expressive language disorders

Overall, cognitive impairments represent a significant impairment for those affected due to their strong influence on psychosocial functioning, but they are often neglected in psychotherapy.

Deficits in cognitive skills can be improved through regular practice. The methods of cognitive remediation mentioned above are a good way of doing this, and intensive training using computer-based programs can be particularly helpful. However, it is even more important that patients practice their cognitive skills in everyday life. There are suggestions for this in Sect. 7.1 (cognitive training).

As those affected find it difficult to concentrate and think, they tend to avoid such situations or give up quickly. In therapy, strategies can be taught that make it possible to work on a task for longer. These include taking breaks, dividing work into small sections, regular study times, and to-do lists.

Neuropsychological tests can be helpful in determining the cognitive strengths of individual patients. As a result, a patient whose verbal memory is impaired while visual perception processing works better, for example, could be taught appropriate learning strategies.

If cognitive training is used, it is worth repeating neuropsychological testing in the course of the treatment to see whether, and in which areas, improvements have occurred.

Therapeutic Conversation with Michael

Michael:	Studying has become so frustrating for me. It's hardly possible anymore. That's why I did almost nothing last week. Then, on Friday, I had two important exams. I must have really messed them up.
Therapist:	I'm sorry to hear that. I know that you've been saying for a long time that your concentration has gotten worse, that you think more slowly, and that you're flooded with so many thoughts at once that you can no longer think clearly.
Michael:	Exactly. You just can't do anything with a head like that. Studying really doesn't do anything for me anymore.
Therapist:	And here in the session, I see you as very clear and focused, someone who thinks quickly and effectively.
Michael:	Sure, but at home it's completely different.
Therapist:	All of the time? Thinking is always so difficult?
Michael:	No, not all the time. But sometimes, I can't concentrate for very long.
Therapist:	How long is it possible for you to concentrate on your work?
Michael:	Hm, maybe 30 minutes at a time on a good day. But then I definitely need a break.
Therapist:	But 30 minutes is already a lot.
Michael:	Yes, but sometimes I feel so exhausted afterwards that I can't remember anything at all.
Therapist:	Studying for 30 minutes is already a very good achievement. If you managed to do something for school for 30 minutes every day, what do you think your school performance would be like?
Michael:	Hm, I would say better.
Therapist:	You're absolutely right, there are good days and bad days. The goal is to keep at it. Even if you can only study for 30 minutes with difficulty, that's already great progress. The chance that you'll manage another 30 minutes the next day increases. Just like with sport, it's the same with thinking: Regular training helps. Keeping at it even on bad days helps you to be in even better shape on the good days. Of course, in addition to the bad days, there are also disaster days. How about giving yourself two joker days a week, when you don't have to do any brain training? On the other five days, however, you could study for 30 minutes a day.
Michael:	And twice a week, I don't have to do anything?
Therapist:	Yes, it's okay that twice a week you don't learn anything. You still can, of course, but you don't have to.
Michael:	And on the other five days I have to?
Therapist:	Let's put it this way: On the other five days, you give it your all to make it work with 30 minutes of studying a day.

5.2.3.2 Delusions

Delusions lead to a misjudgment of reality. The development of delusions is a process in which non-delusional beliefs and fears turn into delusional ideas. Those affected develop beliefs that do not correspond to reality. They cling to their ideas and are not dissuaded by statements from third parties or evidence to the contrary.

Delusions must be distinguished from other thought disorders, such as overvalued ideas or obsessive thoughts, which may appear similar but differ from a delusion in that the affected person is aware that their imposing thoughts and actions do not correspond to reality.

Typical examples of delusional symptoms are:

- So-called first rank symptoms: the feeling that someone or something is controlling one's own thoughts, in the sense of thought insertion, thought interference, external control, or telepathy.
- The feeling of being followed.
- Grandiose ideas.
- Conspiracy theories that can affect the individual or the whole world.
- Nihilistic ideas, i.e., that the world does not really exist and everything is just an illusion.

Treating delusions requires a lot of patience. Delusional ideas are often resistant to treatment, and even medication with antipsychotics sometimes fails to improve the delusional symptoms. An open therapeutic approach is essential. It is less about convincing patients that they are wrong with their paranoid ideas and more about helping them to explore which way of thinking would be most helpful for them at the moment. On the one hand, this process involves working through important life events, current and past, as delusional ideas are often linked to past stressors and learning experiences. On the other hand, the patient's values and belief system should be explored in detail. It is worth spending a lot of time on this. The family background, particularly with regard to religion, politics, or world events, should also be probed in order to gain a detailed picture of how the patient was brought up and the context in which they operate. The next step is to work with patients to identify unfavorable cognitions that contribute to their paranoid beliefs. Various research studies have demonstrated links between abnormalities in social information processing and delusions. The next chapter will go into more detail about the cognitive biases that reinforce delusional thoughts.

It is sometimes difficult for therapists to judge whether certain beliefs are actually delusions, as certain delusional narratives can sound very realistic. In adolescents meeting CHR criteria, the delusions are usually not completely absurd, both in terms of the description and the content, e.g., bullying by schoolmates. It is important not to immediately accuse the patient of delusions but to first ask the parents or teachers how they assess the situation. An objective reality check is practically never possible and is also not the therapist's task.

Instead of speaking out directly against the delusional thoughts, the therapist should validate the patient's stories and perceptions without confirming the delusional beliefs: "I believe you that this situation seemed strange to you and scared you. I have the impression that you are a very intelligent, sensible young person, and I can see that you are convinced that this is what actually happened. But as I wasn't there and only heard your version of the story, I can't say what really happened that night. It could all just be a strange coincidence. I don't know myself. What do you think? How certain are you, in percentage terms, that your interpretation of the situation is correct?"

An important factor in distinguishing between delusions and CHR symptoms is whether patients are still able, at least temporarily, to question their thoughts and respond to external objections. In the CHR stage, most patients are open to looking for alternative explanations for their delusional thoughts. They also experience their paranoid thoughts as very stressful and alienating. This is precisely why these thoughts can cause a great deal of stress. For example, patients are aware that no one can control their thoughts and that it is not possible for them to be fed thoughts by others. It is more of an "as if" feeling and at the same time, leads to great fear of losing control and going crazy. In therapy, young people should be supported in dealing with their insecurity. It is important to discuss in detail with patients what these thoughts trigger in them. Once again, working with the "thoughts-feelings-behavior" triangle is helpful here. The aim is to understand the emotions that trigger these thoughts and the behaviors that patients show in reaction to these thoughts. As in anxiety disorders, avoidance behavior is often observed. For example, patients who feel persecuted will no longer go out alone. As a result of such avoidant safety behavior, alternative experiences that speak against the paranoid ideas are not experienced.

An important part of the treatment is to develop coping strategies with the patient for dealing with these moments. This is not just about changing the paranoid thoughts, but also about managing the stress that these thoughts cause. The coping strategies provided on the worksheet "Paranoid Thoughts" focus primarily on questioning paranoid thoughts and recognizing that they are not real. More information on this can be found in Chap. 6. The last point listed under the strategies is distraction. Other strategies pertaining to the areas of hallucinations, derealization, depersonalization, and anxiety are also useful for managing the stress of these moments. It is worth discussing each strategy with patients and working out what would be helpful for them to cope with the stress they are experiencing in moments of paranoid ideas.

Therapeutic Conversation with Lucy

Lucy:	Yesterday at school, we had a discussion about mental illness. It was awful. Suddenly, I had the feeling that everyone could see that I had mental health problems, and I was afraid that they would know that I was coming here for therapy. The moment I thought about it, I was sure again that the others would be able to hear exactly what I was thinking and really know.
Therapist:	Oh, that sounds extremely unpleasant. What did you do in that situation?
Lucy:	I tried not to think about anything at all. Which of course didn't work. Then I tried to think of something neutral. About lunch, about the fact that I was eating spaghetti.
Therapist:	So, did that work?
Lucy:	Well, at that moment, I realized how silly my assumption was and that, of course, the others couldn't hear my thoughts. That's when I calmed down again.
Therapist:	So, you managed to question and dissolve your assumptions yourself?
Lucy:	Yes. In this situation, yes. I actually know that nobody can hear my thoughts. But in those moments, I'm no longer sure.
Therapist:	Is the strategy of thinking about something else always as helpful as it was yesterday?
Lucy:	No. when I have the feeling that others could hear or read my thoughts, the first thing I always try to do is not think about anything at all, but that usually doesn't work, and I panic. I feel pressure.
Therapist:	And what do you do then?

Lucy:	Sometimes I try desperately to think about something unimportant and trivial, like lunch. That usually makes me realize how absurd my thoughts are. But sometimes I still don't. In those moments, the fear remains that others will hear what I'm thinking and judge me for it. And then I can see it on their faces.
Therapist:	How do you manage to get away from these thoughts and the stress that is caused by them?
Lucy:	I try to take a deep breath. Very slowly. Just like I learned in therapy: Inhale and exhale deeply three times, then slightly push my legs into the floor as I exhale. This helps me to calm down a little. As soon as I get away from these panic-like sensations, I can think a bit more clearly again. Then, at some point, I manage to tell myself how absurd my idea that others could hear or read my thoughts is.
Therapist:	It seems to me you've already made a lot of progress. Are there any other things that you try that help you?
Lucy:	When it gets really bad, I chew gum. Then I think no one can hear my thoughts if I chew loudly enough. I know that sounds stupid. I also feel stupid saying something like that. Like I'm a real psycho who chews gum so that nobody can hear her thoughts.
Therapist:	Lucy, that's not stupid. You've realized that it's important for you to calm down in those moments. As soon as you can calm down, you'll be able to question your thoughts again. Just not when you're so upset. So, if chewing gum helps you in those really difficult moments, it's a great strategy.
Lucy:	It's just that I'm kind of ashamed. That I keep coming up with these irrational ideas.
Therapist:	The way you describe it, it seems to happen in moments that are very stressful for you. As soon as the stress decreases slightly, you can think more clearly again. I think it's important that you have recognized this and are actively doing something to reduce the stress at these times.

5.3 Comorbid Symptoms

As already mentioned at the beginning of the book, most patients who come in for consultation also show other comorbid symptoms in addition to the so-called CHR symptoms.

Most frequently reported are depressive symptoms, which have already been discussed in the chapter on alterations in mood and drive. In addition, patients often report difficulties concentrating, which may be related to the CHR status but may also be the result of depression or comorbid ADHD.

Other typical comorbid symptoms reported by adolescents meeting CHR are anxiety, sleep problems, and substance abuse. These three symptoms are discussed in more detail below.

5.3.1 Anxiety

Patients meeting CHR criteria report symptoms of anxiety. Although CHR symptoms themselves can cause severe anxiety, often including panic attacks, many patients with CHR symptoms show a comorbid anxiety disorder that was present before the onset of CHR symptoms.

Anxiety should be explored in detail with all adolescents with CHR symptoms.

As anxiety is a potentially embarrassing topic, especially for adolescents, they should be asked about it repeatedly during the course of treatment. It may take several sessions before patients feel comfortable talking about it.

Cognitive behavioral therapy is the treatment of choice for anxiety disorders, as it has been shown to be highly successful. In the following, the psychotherapeutic treatment of anxiety will not be discussed in detail, as this would exceed the scope of this book; only some important points regarding the treatment of anxiety symptoms in adolescents with CHR symptoms will be presented.

5.3.1.1 Panic Disorders

Perceptive disturbances are a particularly common cause of panic in patients meeting CHR criteria. Besides concerns about hallucinatory or paranoid ideas per se, many patients express a general worry about going crazy and losing control. Psychoeducation about the CHR symptoms themselves and coping strategies for dealing with them can provide some relief and reduce panic.

It is important to communicate to patients that experiencing anxiety in response to the CHR symptoms is a normal reaction.

If the anxiety symptoms persist, it is worth working on better ways of dealing with the panic itself. The following strategies are recommended:

- Detailed psychoeducation on the biological background of anxiety symptoms and explanation of the vicious cycle of anxiety
- Cognitive restructuring of anxiety to identify and challenge unhelpful thoughts
- Strategies to relax, ground, and distract

5.3.1.2 Social Phobia

A very common diagnosis in adolescents with CHR symptoms is social phobia, which can develop over time into distrust and persecutory ideation. In these cases, it is important to treat social anxiety according to established guidelines for social phobia.

Overall, the topic of social interactions and skills should play a major role in the therapy with young people meeting CHR criteria. Many adolescents feel more insecure in their social interactions than before and report a marked social withdrawal. Others say that they have always been loners and that social contact is not particularly important to them. The therapist should still pursue work on social skills, even in the presence of such statements. Contact with peers is extremely important in childhood and especially in adolescence. Strengthening social skills is essential in terms of prevention, as a lack of social skills is associated with a higher risk of developing psychosis.

In addition to individual therapy focused on social skills, group training sessions are also effective. At our early intervention center in Zurich, we have group therapy for patients meeting CHR criteria, in which social skills training plays an important role. However, patients can also benefit from less specific social skills training that is not explicitly aimed at patients meeting CHR criteria. The advantage of group training is the direct feedback from peers, which enhances the transfer of skills to everyday life. The group dynamic reflects real-life situations more effectively than the individual sessions with the therapist.

5.3.1.3 Specific Phobia

Patients with CHR symptoms often report new, specific phobias that have developed recently. In therapy, the thoughts behind these new fears and whether they are related to the experience of CHR symptoms should be explored in detail. For example, a fear of the dark is often described as being caused by the experience of CHR symptoms (fear of persecution, hallucinations, and illusory misperceptions that occur mainly at night). If this is the case, it can be assumed that the fear will decrease if the risk symptoms are treated.

In the case of a defined specific phobia, it is necessary to assess the degree of interference with daily life and the level of distress. Based on this assessment, therapy for the phobia may be recommended. However, if other problems are more important, treatment of the phobia may be deferred to a later stage.

5.3.1.4 Generalized Anxiety Disorder

In generalized anxiety disorder, anxiety is not focused on specific stimuli but is free-floating, with potentially any aspect of daily life being perceived as threatening.

Here, a distinction needs to be drawn as to whether the generalized anxiety has arisen as a result of the CHR symptoms or the other way around. The CHR symptoms change the perceived environment and can create high levels of uncertainty, which can lead to generalized anxiety disorder. In this case, the anxiety should decrease if the risk symptoms are treated. Conversely, CHR symptoms may develop as a result of generalized anxiety. The higher stress of daily life caused by anxiety increases vulnerability to risk symptoms. In this case, it is likely that CHR symptoms will decrease if the patient learns better coping strategies for anxiety.

5.3.2 Sleep Problems

In any case, sleep hygiene should be an important part of the management of patients who meet the CHR criteria. Sleep problems can have a significant impact on coping with daily life, and sleep deprivation can increase vulnerability to stress. Addressing sleep problems is also important in order to prevent self-medication with sleep-inducing substances such as cannabis or alcohol. As sleep deprivation is associated with the development of psychosis, treating comorbid sleep problems helps to prevent the transition to psychosis.

Advice on improving sleep quality (see worksheet “Sleep Problems”) should be discussed in detail with patients. However, it should also be noted that some patients may still report significant sleep disturbance despite adherence to sleep hygiene practices. In such cases, pharmacological treatment of the sleep problem, such as valerian or melatonin, should be considered to help the patient establish a regular sleep-wake cycle.

5.3.3 Substance Abuse

Treating the use of illegal or legal substances is a very high priority. Motivation to stop using is one of the most important factors in a successful therapeutic alliance.

Many patients meeting CHR criteria use substances to self-medicate. Although substances such as cannabis can aggravate or even trigger symptoms, it is also possible for symptoms to decrease when intoxicated. However, as soon as the effects wear off, the symptoms return, sometimes more severely than before. To address this aspect, it is recommended that the therapist discuss whether a medication that provides a similar but more sustained symptom-relieving effect would be more appropriate than the current substances.

Depending on the extent of substance abuse, counseling in a specialized substance abuse center may be an option in addition to the therapy.

5.3.3.1 Illegal Drugs

There has been a debate over the years as to whether cannabis and other drugs can trigger psychosis or whether the association between the use of illegal substances and psychosis is due to the fact that these patients use drugs more than the general population as a form of self-medication. In our experience at the Early Intervention Center, cannabis in particular can often trigger risk symptoms (e.g., visual hallucinations, derealization and depersonalization, or paranoid thoughts). Whether these symptoms would have occurred in the absence of cannabis use cannot ultimately be determined. Patients need to be fully informed about the relationship between psychosis and drug use. Therapists should encourage complete abstinence from all substance use.

At the same time, therapists should be aware of the impact that complete withdrawal from all substances can have on young people. Cannabis, in particular, is often part of the youth culture. Resisting the constant temptation is a major challenge. In addition to the desire to get high, young people have to withstand strong peer pressure. Therefore, it should be all the more recognized as a major achievement for the patient to give up drugs completely.

A clear agreement with patients that they cannot attend appointments under the influence of drugs is an important prerequisite for successful treatment. Patients who turn up on drugs must be sent home, and a new appointment should be arranged.

Nevertheless, a moralizing attitude towards substance use is not helpful for the therapeutic relationship. Instead, the therapist should discuss the effects, side effects, and risks of drugs openly, neutrally, and repeatedly. Individual motives for substance use need to be explored in detail. During the therapy session, a list of pros and cons should be drawn up, including both short- and long-term effects. Many patients use drugs as a coping strategy to improve their mood or forget their problems. This underlines the importance of working with patients to identify alternative strategies that achieve similar desired effects in a more adaptive way.

Immediate abstinence is not always realistic, so gradual reduction can be a big success. Keep in mind that the word "relapse" is generally stigmatizing and not very helpful. It is more helpful to talk about a "single event" after using it again. Then, discuss openly with the patient how it happened and what could be done differently next time.

Abstinence can lead to a loss of social connections and friendships. Finding a new circle of friends is a major challenge. Therapists should remain aware of this and explore how friends respond to the patient's attempts at abstinence.

5.3.3.2 Alcohol

Fortunately, daily alcohol consumption is less common in adolescent patients than in adult psychiatry.

Despite this, many adolescents with CHR symptoms already show problematic use of alcohol. In particular, many young people who have previously consumed cannabis turn to alcohol instead once their CHR status has been established, as they perceive it to have a lower risk of triggering psychosis.

A similar therapeutic approach is recommended for alcohol use as for the use of illegal substances. The risks and dangers of regular alcohol consumption need to be explained objectively, especially the interaction between medication and alcohol.

Many young people report that they drink to forget their problems. Talking to them about what they could be doing instead is therefore a key factor in the treatment.

Demonizing alcohol makes little sense in therapy. Especially as alcohol consumption is not usually stigmatized in Western societies. Aiming for a moderate approach can be a goal of therapy, especially to prevent excessive relapse, such as thinking, "I've already had a beer, so it doesn't matter now anyway!"

5.4 Protocols

In order to determine the relationship between internal factors and external events (including the time of day) and symptoms, and to gain a better overview of the extent of symptoms, it is important that patients keep a diary of how they feel. Daily logging of mood and symptoms is particularly recommended during the assessment phase and at the start of treatment. Several log templates are included in this book.

5.4.1 Mood Protocols

The use of mood protocols is useful at different stages of treatment. During the diagnostic phase, protocols provide a better idea of possible mood swings and depressive and manic symptoms. It is recommended that the logs be completed over several weeks to get as accurate a picture as possible. Typical daily fluctuations, such as a drop in mood towards the evening, as well as weekly fluctuations, such as a worsening of mood towards the end of the week, may become apparent. Patients are often unaware of these patterns. Many patients report that they feel bad all the time and that their mood rarely improves. Mood diaries can provide a more realistic picture.

Therapeutic Conversation with Michael

Therapist:	You yourself often describe how you feel like your mood swings come out of nowhere and that you can't understand the reasons for them. But if we take a closer look at your mood logs over the last few weeks, I notice a few patterns. Do you too?
Michael:	Yes, overall, my mood usually gets worse in the middle of the week.
Therapist:	Exactly, I see a downward trend from Wednesday onwards. On the other hand, your mood improves again on Saturday and Sunday. Can you think of anything off the top of your head that could explain this pattern?
Michael:	We have a vocational school all day on Wednesday. That's exhausting for me. I have to concentrate all day, and I often feel overwhelmed by the school material. If we also get exams back that aren't good, I'm really demotivated.
Therapist:	That's understandable. What do you do in the evening after such an intense day?
Michael:	Actually, I always plan to study a lot and repeat everything we've learned that day. But often I don't make any progress at all and end up doing nothing.
Therapist:	And how does that make you feel?
Michael:	You can see on the mood log: On Wednesday evenings, my mood is usually in the basement. I can't even go to sleep afterwards because I'm worried about my apprenticeship. Then I come to work on Thursday, overtired and unmotivated.
Therapist:	If we look at your mood log and look at the moments when you feel good, what do you notice? When are these?
Michael:	When I meet my friends I feel good. So, the weekends. And on Monday evenings, at football training.
Therapist:	So whenever you do an activity that you enjoy?
Michael:	You could say that, yes.
Therapist:	On Wednesday, after vocational school, wouldn't it be good if you did something fun? For example, meeting a friend?
Michael:	For my mood, yes. But my conscience... Is rather difficult. I would think that I had to go home to study.
Therapist:	I see it like this: You are exhausted after a whole day at school and hardly have any energy left to study. You're trying anyway, which shows me that you're very motivated in your studies, but it's not necessarily helpful. Especially given that you're so worried afterwards that you can't sleep well. If, on the other hand, you end the day doing a more positive activity and your mood improves by a few points, then I imagine that it could be easier for you to fall asleep. Don't you think so?
Michael:	Probably yes.
Therapist:	And how do you think that will affect your mood on Thursday morning?
Michael:	It'll probably be a bit better.

Mood logs are also useful for measuring progress. Pre-therapy logs can be compared with logs after a few weeks of therapy, and patients can be shown progress. It is always advisable to submit a mood log when starting medication.

The worksheets contain four different types of mood logs. The first one asks patients to rate their mood on a scale of 0–10 four times a day.

Many adolescents find it difficult to rate their mood using a number. In these cases, the second mood log can be used. Similar to a traffic light system, patients can mark their mood between red (I feel very bad) and green (I feel very good). The third worksheet also uses colors and is used to record possible depressive or (hypo-) manic symptoms if bipolar disorder is suspected. Both low and high moods can be colored red. However, a scale from −10 to 10, which could also be helpful in identifying bipolar mood swings, has been deliberately omitted. Keeping mood diaries has a direct effect on the patient's state of mind; describing one's own state of mind in the negative range can cause the mood to worsen.

Not only at the time of recording, but also in retrospect, a weekly log with many entries in the minus range has a discouraging effect. Of course, a mood log with all the information in the red zone also has a negative effect. However, the authors suggest that a color scheme is less frustrating than a numerical negative range.

The final worksheet on mood is designed to help patients themselves better understand the relationship between behavior and mood. Patients should actively try to improve their mood. The list of positive activities (in the Robin Z app or the worksheets in Sect. 7.6) is a good way of doing this. They should choose one activity per day and assess their mood before and after the activity. This type of mood diary helps to increase feelings of self-efficacy about one's mental state.

Mood and Symptom Protocols

Clinical experience has shown that mood and symptom diaries are filled out only occasionally and that patients often forget to bring them to therapy sessions. It is also not realistic for patients to carry their paper diaries with them at all times, which makes real-time recording difficult. For this and other reasons, the Robin Z app was developed. Symptoms and mood, as well as any other events, can be documented directly in the app's logbook. Under Settings, patients can set reminders for their logbook entries.

In the tutorial video "Logbook" (Fig. 5.3), therapists are given tips and instructions on how to use the logbook in **therapy sessions.**

There is a tutorial video "**Reminders**" (Fig. 5.4) for setting the reminder function.

A graphical representation of the logbook data is possible with the analysis program Robin View, details of which can be found in the tutorial videos "**Share My Data**" (Fig. 5.5) and "Robin View" (Fig. 5.6).

5.4.2 Symptom Protocols

There are two samples of symptom log sheets among the worksheets. The first symptom log is used to record individual symptoms over the course of a week. It is up to the adolescent to decide whether to record the intensity of each symptom,

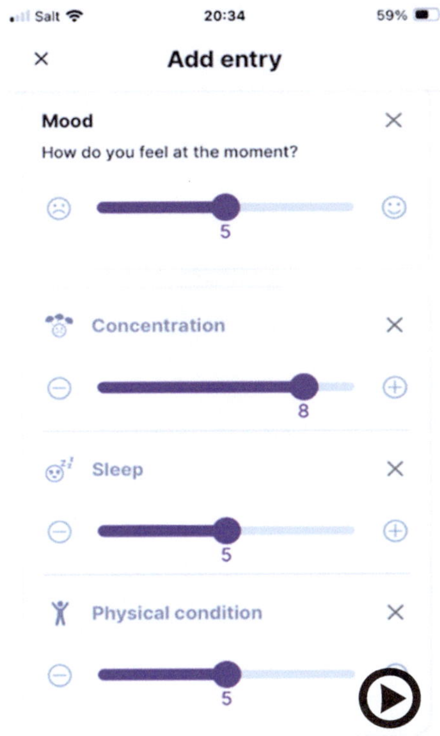

Fig. 5.3 Tutorial video "Logbook" (▶ https://doi.org/10.1007/000-k5f)

the frequency of each symptom per day, or simply whether the symptom is present or not by ticking the boxes. Therefore, the log can be filled in daily without much effort.

The second worksheet, "Dealing With My Symptoms," is recommended for more detailed recording and observation of individual symptoms. Here, the circumstances in which the symptoms occurred and their intensity are recorded. At the same time, the coping strategies used and their effectiveness are recorded. This encourages patients to take an active role in managing their symptoms.

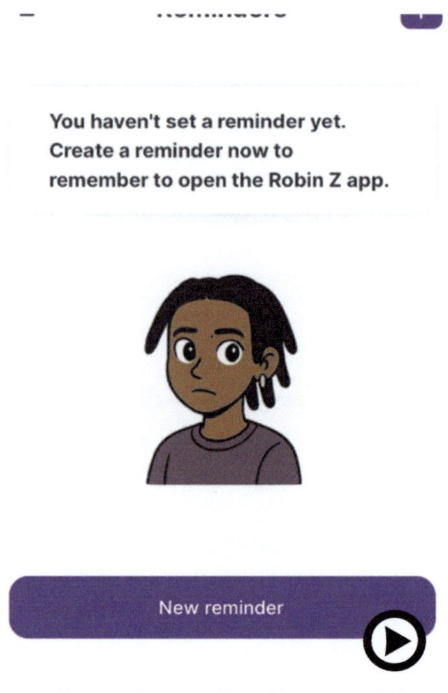
You haven't set a reminder yet.
Create a reminder now to
remember to open the Robin Z app.
New reminder

Fig. 5.4 Tutorial video "Reminders" (▶ https://doi.org/10.1007/000-k5e)

Therapeutic Conversation with Lucy

Therapist:	Last week you kept a record of your irritability, anxiety, sleep, concentration, and hallucinations. Did you notice anything when filling it in?
Lucy:	Hm, I think it's all to do with my sleep problems. If I don't sleep well, I'm tired during the day and can't concentrate well. I'm also much more irritable.
Therapist:	Yes, I see that, too. There's a connection in your statements. And of course it's the same for everyone. If we sleep badly and are tired, we can't concentrate well and are more irritable.
Lucy:	Yes, I'm naturally more irritable because I'm tired. But I get even more irritable because I can't concentrate. I get angry with myself and frustrated, which makes things worse.
Therapist:	That also explains why your irritability increases throughout the day.
Lucy:	*(nods)*
Therapist:	Do you have more hallucinations when you haven't slept well the night before?
Lucy:	The hallucinations are actually always there. But when I'm more irritable, I can't handle it well.
Therapist:	Does that mean the hallucinations are also there on good days?
Lucy:	Yes, but then I just ignore them. I don't pay attention to them, so then they disappear again.
Therapist:	If I understand correctly, you are saying that sleep problems have a negative effect on concentration and irritability. When you sleep badly, you are more irritable, and when you are more irritable, you experience the hallucinations as more stressful.
Lucy:	Exactly, and I can't ignore them either. I can distract myself less, so they bother me all the more.

Therapist:	So the more irritable you are, the less able you are to deal with the hallucinations?
Lucy:	Exactly.
Therapist:	Does the reverse also apply? That your hallucinations influence your irritability?
Lucy:	*(thinks for a moment)* of course the hallucinations annoy me, and I sometimes get a bit angry. But actually, I think they scare me more. And when I'm scared, they get stronger. And when they go away, I'm afraid they'll come back. I often can't sleep well in the evening because I'm afraid I might have hallucinations. Oh, it's all connected somehow...
Therapist:	You're right about that. But I'd like to come back to the fact that you said at the beginning that your sleep problems were at the heart of the matter. Perhaps we can take that up again: Do you think that if we could get a better handle on your sleep problems, it would have a positive impact on your other issues?
Lucy:	Probably yes. I would be less tired and less irritable and could concentrate better. I could deal with the hallucinations better and wouldn't be so afraid.

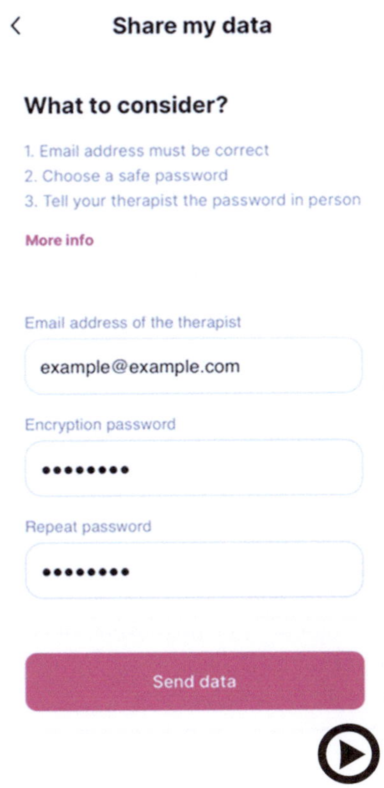

Fig. 5.5 Tutorial video "Share My Data" (▶ https://doi.org/10.1007/000-k5h)

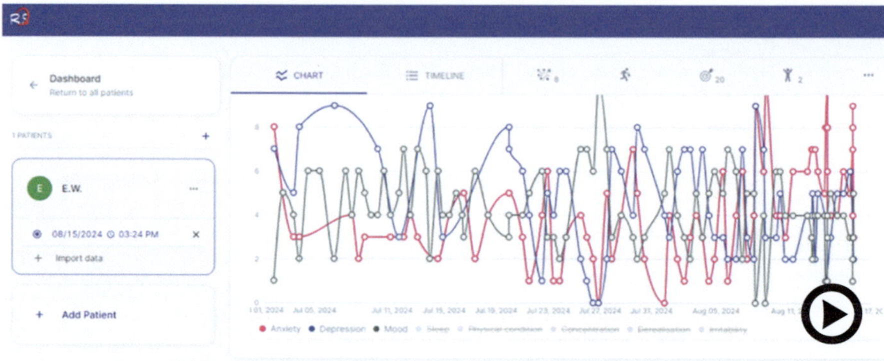

Fig. 5.6 Tutorial video "Robin View" (▶ https://doi.org/10.1007/000-k5j)

5.5 Worksheets

The following worksheets (see Fig. 5.7) belong to this chapter and are available online for download in the context of the electronic chapter:

- Worksheet 13 "Depression"
- Worksheet 14 "Elated Feelings"
- Worksheet 15 "Irritability"
- Worksheet 16 "Derealization and Depersonalization"
- Worksheet 17 "Hallucinations"
- Worksheet 18 "Hearing Voices"
- Worksheet 19 "Concentration Problems"
- Worksheet 20 "Thought Disturbances"
- Worksheet 21 "Delusion"
- Worksheet 22 "Anxiety"
- Worksheet 23 "Sleeping Problems"
- Worksheet 24 "Substance Use"
- Worksheets 25–27 "Mood Protocol"
- Worksheets 28 and 29 "Protocol of Positive Activities"
- Worksheet 30 "Symptom Protocol"
- Worksheet 31 "Dealing with Symptoms"

Depression

Depression often appears as a persistent feeling of sadness, loss of energy, inner emptiness, or even hopelessness. Physical symptoms such as sleep problems, loss of appetite, or excessive tiredness are common. It is important to remember that depression is not your fault. Depression is an illness with different symptoms that affect your thoughts, emotions, body, and behaviour.

The vicious circle of depression:

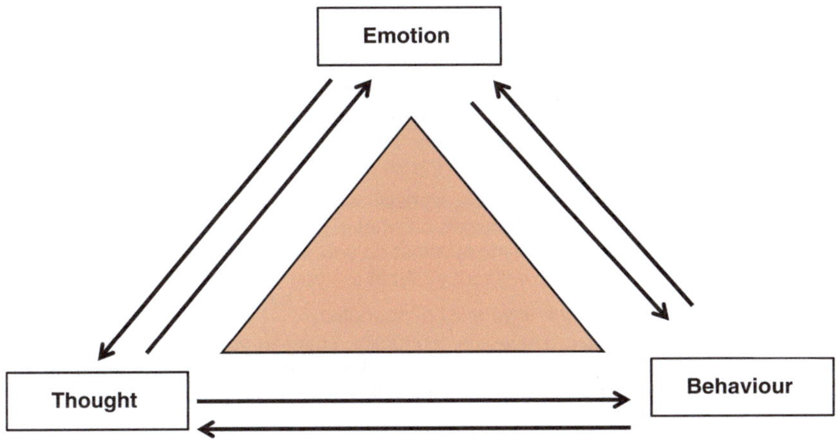

Depression often leads to depressive behaviours such as staying in bed, withdrawing from others, and becoming less active. These behaviours are often accompanied by negative thoughts such as "I'm a total loser".

Emotions, behaviour, and thoughts are all connected. How we feel is linked to how we behave and what we think. That's why we can change our feelings by changing our behaviour or thinking.

It can be helpful to reframe negative thoughts and focus on more positive ones. For example, instead of thinking "I can't do anything", try recognising small successes. Even small activities like going for a walk or talking to friends can help break the negative cycle and improve your mood.

Fig. 5.7 Worksheet 13 to Worksheet 31

Depression

Tips for dealing with depression:

- ✓ **Positive activities:** Even just five minutes spent on an enjoyable activity can make a difference (see worksheet "Positive Activities").
- ✓ **Stop thinking:** Negative thoughts, self-blame, and guilt are not helpful. When these thoughts come over you, say politely and kindly to yourself: "Stop. This isn't helpful."
- ✓ **Self-encouragement:** Ask yourself, what would you say to a good friend or someone you like in your family who is going through the same thing? How would you try to cheer them up and encourage them?
- ✓ **Fair perspective:** Thoughts like "I have to" or "I should" can create unnecessary pressure. In moments when you're not feeling well, remember: you don't have to and you don't need to push yourself beyond what you're capable of.
- ✓ **Check your expectations:** You are not at your best right now, and it is therefore normal that you cannot meet all your expectations. Remember, you wouldn't try to climb a mountain with a broken leg. It's the same with your depression.
- ✓ **What is going well?:** We tend to have a pessimistic mindset, especially when we are not feeling well. Counter this by focusing on what is going well at the moment. Take a look at your list of positive experiences. What do you like about yourself, others, and your environment? What went well today? What are you grateful for?
- ✓ **List of Strength:** Take a look at your list of strengths.
- ✓ **Check your body posture:** There is a connection between our posture and how we feel. An upright, open body posture can help us feel more optimistic and powerful. Check your body alignment. Try to keep your back straight and your shoulders relaxed. Also: chest out, stomach in, and head up.
- ✓ **Smiling can improve your mood:** Sometimes just smiling can lift your mood. Our brain sends signals to our muscles to smile when we're happy, but it also works the other way around. Smiling can signal to your brain that you're happy and make you feel happy, even if you don't feel like smiling at first.
- ✓ **Get outside:** Fresh air and daylight have a mood-lifting effect. Even if it takes some effort, a short walk around the block can improve your mood.
- ✓ **Relaxation exercises:** Try one of the relaxation exercises from the worksheet "Positive Activities". Relaxation helps to promote positive thinking.
- ✓ **Do the opposite:** Depression is not a good counsellor. Your current impulses and ideas aren't helpful for you. Do the opposite of what your depression wants you to do. For example, if your impulse is to go back to bed and hide, try taking a shower and then getting some fresh air. If you don't feel like talking to anyone, pick up your phone and text at least three people.
- ✓ **Daily self-care:** When you're not feeling well, it's important to take care of your basic needs. Only when these are met will your mood begin to improve. Make sure you get enough (but not too much) sleep (see the worksheet "Sleep Problems"). Try to keep up with your hygiene routine, such as brushing your teeth, showering, and combing your

Fig. 5.7 (continued)

hair. Make sure you eat regularly, even if you have little appetite. Try to eat at least three meals a day.

✓ **Talk about it:** Sometimes it helps to talk to someone about how you're feeling. Writing down your feelings, perhaps in a journal or diary, can also help. Paper is patient and doesn't judge.

✓ **Energy balance:** Don't overextend yourself right now. It's important to use your energy wisely. Do only what absolutely needs to be done today; everything else can wait.

✓ **Feelings are temporary.** No emotion lasts a lifetime. Just as it's impossible to feel happy all the time, it's also impossible to feel sad and down forever. Right now it may feel like your mood will never improve, that's not the case. Every emotion is a temporary state. It can last a long time, but it is a feeling, it will pass. Even if you feel depressed, look at your mood diary - aren't there fluctuations? Moments when you felt at least a little better?

✓ **Don't wait for better feelings:** Don't wait until you feel more energetic, motivated, or even cheerful. Just do it anyway. Feelings of happiness or energy may follow, even after you've started.

✓ **Question your automatic thoughts:** Many thoughts happen so quickly that we don't consciously notice them. These thought patterns are called automatic thoughts, and each of us has them. They're useful in everyday life because it would be overwhelming to actively think about every single thing all the time. But automatic thoughts can also worsen our mood without us knowing exactly why. Try to work with your therapist to identify the automatic thought patterns you tend to use. Together, you can look for strategies to recognise and question negative thought patterns.

✓ **Maintain a daily structure:** Sometimes, when we feel very low, we may not feel like doing anything, even getting out of bed. But if we follow these impulses, our mental well-being will get worse, not better. It's important to stick to a daily routine and continue to go to school or work every day. If your work or school routine feels overwhelming, be sure to discuss this with your therapist so that your daily structure can be adjusted to your condition if necessary.

Own Ideas:

✓ …

✓ …

✓ …

Fig. 5.7 (continued)

Elated Feelings

We all hope that things will go well in our lives, and that we'll feel happy. Sometimes, however, you may feel overly positive and have so much energy that it can actually be uncomfortable. You may feel that you do not need to sleep, or that you have a lot of ideas in your head that you need to talk about very quickly. Others may also complain about your behaviour. Because of this feeling of elation, you may do things that are dangerous and risky, such as spending more money than you have. These extreme feelings of elation are called hypomania or manic phases.

When you recognise these feelings of elation, it is very important that you talk about them in a therapy session. Together, you and your therapist can discuss how to prevent or at least minimise the negative effects of these episodes.

It's also important that you learn to recognise early warning signs. Discuss with your therapist what the triggers are and what the first symptom(s) look like.

Tips for dealing with elated feelings:

- ✓ **List of warning signs:** React as soon as you notice any of the warning signs. Get in touch with your therapist.
- ✓ **Relaxation exercises:** Refer to the worksheet "Positive Activities" for relaxation ideas. If possible, try relaxation exercises once a day – even ten minutes can help.
- ✓ **No substance use:** Stay away from all drugs and avoid excessive caffeine.
- ✓ **Daily routine:** Aim for a structured daily routine with regular sleep times (always around the same time), regular meals, and also a regular daily structure with school, work and leisure activities.
- ✓ **Avoid overstimulation:** Don't take on too much.
- ✓ **Mood diary:** Track your mood several times a day in a mood diary. Along with your mood, record factors like sleep, substance use, or any stressful experiences. Tracking your mood can help you identify patterns in when these highs tend to occur.
- ✓ **Slow down your impulsive reactions:** Be aware of your impulses and ideas, as they may not be helpful at the moment. Question and evaluate each one.
- ✓ **Withdraw:** In moments when you feel overly driven, consider stepping back and doing something quiet, such as listening to calming music, taking a warm bath, or drinking a warm herbal tea.

Fig. 5.7 (continued)

✓ **Avoid multitasking:** Tasks that require frequent switching between activities can increase these feelings. Focus on one task at a time and work through routine activities slowly and consciously. Try to give your full attention to one thing at a time.

✓ **Rethink your decisions:** In moments of high energy, we tend to make impulsive or very decisions, such as overspending. Avoid rash decisions by giving yourself time to think about each decision before you make it.

✓ **Protective measures:** Take steps to protect yourself from the potential negative effects of these highs. For example, if you tend to overspend, consider lowering your monthly credit card limit.

Own Ideas:

✓ ...

✓ ...

✓ ...

Fig. 5.7 (continued)

Irritability

We all have moments when we feel irritable, tense or emotional. During these times, even small things and unimportant events can trigger intense reactions, such as exploding, ranting, or suddenly starting to cry.

Sometimes our irritability has specific reasons - such as lack of sleep, stress at school, or family problems. Other times, we may feel irritable for no particular reason; we just wake up in a bad mood. We're often more prone to irritability when we're already feeling low or unwell.

These overreactions can have unwanted consequences, such as hurting or upsetting others with our emotional reactions. Being aware of our irritable moods and taking steps to address them can help us manage these moods better.

Tips for dealing with irritability:

✓ **Be kind to yourself:** When you're feeling tense and irritable, take time to do something good for yourself, like engaging in a pleasant activity (see worksheet "Positive Activities").

✓ **Put a brake on your impulsive reaction:** In these moments, your impulses may not be helpful to you. Question your urges and ideas before you act on them. Being aware of your own irritability is an important step.

✓ **Feelings are temporary:** Emotions such as anger or irritation can feel very intense, but they rarely last long. All emotions are temporary, there is no such thing as a permanent feeling. Remember that emotions come and go; just as we don't feel happy all the time, it's impossible to feel angry forever. So try to be aware and remind yourself that your anger is just a feeling, and it will pass.

✓ **Anger is okay:** It's OK to be angry. Being angry is a sign that some of your needs are being neglected at the moment. See your anger as an important indication of your needs.

✓ **Breathing technique:** If you notice yourself getting more and more upset, stop for a moment and take three deep breaths to calm yourself.

✓ **Spaghetti:** Tense all your muscles and then relax them, releasing built-up tension.

✓ **Anti-Stress ball:** Keep a small stress ball or similar object nearby to squeeze when you feel tense.

✓ **Physical activity:** Channel your anger into physical activity, such as a workout, to release and manage your emotions constructively.

Fig. 5.7 (continued)

- ✓ **Check your posture:** There is an interaction between our posture and our state of mind. Especially when we are tense, we tend to tense up physically. This, in turn, increases our irritability. Check your posture. Try to adopt an open, upright posture.
- ✓ **Relaxation exercises:** Relaxation techniques such as autogenic training, yoga, or progressive muscle relaxation can help reduce irritability. If possible, try to do one of these techniques every day. Five minutes is plenty of time.
- ✓ **Talk about it:** Talking about your anger can be helpful. It is often helpful to talk to a third, uninvolved person. Talk to a friend, colleague, family member, or therapist about how you are feeling.
- ✓ **Withdrawal:** In moments of irritability, it can be helpful to step back and spend some time alone until you have calmed down.
- ✓ **Energy balance:** Don't overdo it. It's important to manage your energy wisely. Focus only on what absolutely has to be done today; everything else can wait.
- ✓ **Eat regularly:** Sometimes there is a very simple reason for irritability, such as hunger. Did you eat enough today?
- ✓ **Make sure you get enough sleep.** If you have trouble sleeping, check out the tips on sleep problems.
- ✓ **No substance use:** Avoid drugs and too much coffee. These tend to make you even more irritable.

- ✓ Own Ideas:

- ✓ …

- ✓ …

- ✓ …

Fig. 5.7 (continued)

Derealisation and Depersonalisation

Derealisation: In derealisation, the environment and other people are experienced as strange and unreal. Everything may seem different, unreal, or fake, as if you are in a film or behind a screen.

Depersonalisation: Depersonalisation is when you experience yourself or your feelings as strange or alien. You may feel as though you're hearing yourself speak from a distance, standing next to yourself, or that everything happens automatically. Your body may feel completely unfamiliar.

Derealisation and depersonalisation are common in young people, especially during stressful times. They don't necessarily indicate psychosis, although they can make you feel like you're losing control or "going mad".

Tips for coping with derealisation and depersonalisation:

- ✓ **Mindfulness exercises:** Focus on small, everyday activities. For instance, concentrate fully on unlocking your front door. Try to consciously pursue this activity with all your concentration and all your senses.
- ✓ **Physical activities:** Any physical activity is very helpful in dealing with these symptoms. It doesn't have to be a marathon. For some suggestions, see the physical activities on the worksheet "Positive Activities".
- ✓ **Hydrotherapy:** Start with warm water, then cold water, then warm water and so on. Focus on how the difference in temperature affects your body.
- ✓ **Drinking:** Mindfully drink a glass of water. Notice the sensations.
- ✓ **Mindful eating:** Focus on the food. How does it taste? What is its consistency? How does it feel when you chew?
- ✓ **Breathing exercise:** Breathe deeply in and out three times.
- ✓ **Petting an animal:** Petting a dog, cat or other animal can be grounding.
- ✓ **Combing your hair:** This simple activity can help you focus on the present moment.
- ✓ **Painting your nails:** Requiring focus and concentration, this activity is a great mindfulness exercise. It also encourages self-care, which can help you feel more connected to yourself.
- ✓ **Walking barefoot:** Feel the ground beneath your feet as a way to reconnect.
- ✓ **Sing out loud**: Expressing yourself vocally can shift your focus and energy.
- ✓ **Social activities:** Feelings of derealisation or depersonalisation often lessen when we are around other people and engage in conversation with someone.
- ✓ **Touching yourself or someone else:** Touch provides direct sensory input and a tangible reminder that you are present in your body and in the real world. This helps to counteract the sense of disconnection.
- ✓ **Pinch yourself:** Pinching yourself can be a useful grounding technique to help you focus on the present moment and reconnect with your body.
- ✓ **Spaghetti:** Tense and then relax all your muscles.

Fig. 5.7 (continued)

- ✓ **Touch**Explore different textures or surfaces to engage your senses.
- ✓ **Brushing your teeth:** Use a strong toothpaste and focus on the sensation.
- ✓ **Balance exercise:** Walking on a straight line is a good mindfulness exercise and can help to centre you.
- ✓ **Stay grounded:** Actively connect with the present moment by touching a wall or a solid, stable object such as a table. Another option is to press your feet into the floor as firmly as possible.
- ✓ **Daily structure:** Create a routine in your daily life with regular bedtimes (always around the same time, to provide enough sleep), regular meals, as well as a daily structure with school, work, and leisure activities.

Own Ideas:

- ✓ …
- ✓ …
- ✓ …

Fig. 5.7 (continued)

Hallucinations

Hallucinations refers to perceiving something that is not actually there. For example, seeing people or animals that others cannot see. Hallucinations can affect any of our senses (hearing, sight, touch, smell, or taste).
They can occur when certain parts of the brain are mistakenly activated. Hallucinations are more common in young people and often disappear on their own.

Tips for dealing with hallucinations:

- ✓ **Reality check:** Keep reminding yourself that it's just your brain playing tricks on you. Look for evidence that your hallucinations can't be real.
- ✓ **Close and open your eyes:** To reset your perception, close your eyes briefly and then open them again.
- ✓ **Relaxation exercises:** You can find suggestions for relaxation exercises in the worksheet "Positive Activities".
- ✓ **Look elsewhere:** Focus your attention somewhere else and then look back.
- ✓ **Send them away:** Send your hallucination away. You can get angry or shout at it.
- ✓ **To ground yourself:** Hallucinations can make you feel detached and drifting away. To counteract this, ground yourself by actively focusing on the present moment. The easiest way to do this is to touch a wall or a fixed, stable object such as a table. Another option is to press your feet into the floor as hard as you can.
- ✓ **Protective wall:** Exclude yourself from your hallucination. Imagine a wall or protective circle around you that the hallucination cannot cross.
- ✓ **Distraction:** Do something to distract yourself, such as something from the list of positive activities.
- ✓ **See through hallucinations:** Keep a log or diary of when and how the hallucinations occur, noting their intensity and the circumstances surrounding them. This may help you to identify patterns in your hallucinations and make them more predictable.
- ✓ **Ask others**Ask others around you if they hear, see, smell, or taste the same thing.
- ✓ **What does hallucination represent?** In psychology we assume that every symptom signifies or represents a need that is not being met sufficiently at the moment. Think about what needs your hallucinations might be pointing to. What might they be trying to tell you?
- ✓ **Ignore them:** Sometimes, despite trying all of the above, the hallucinations may not go away. If this happens, remember that they cannot harm you. You can go about your daily life and they don't have to affect your behaviour.

Own Ideas:

- ✓ …
- ✓ …
- ✓ …

Fig. 5.7 (continued)

Hearing Voices

Sometimes you may hear voices that others cannot hear. This happens when the wrong part of the brain being activated. The part of the brain responsible for speech is falsely activated, so you hear something.

Hearing voices that others don't hear is the most common form of hallucination. It occurs more often than you might think, but very few people talk about it. Studies have shown that up to 20 percent people hear such voices at least once in their lifetime.

Tips for dealing with hearing voices:

✓ **Reality check:** Remind yourself that the voices are not real. It's just your brain playing tricks on you. If there really was a voice, wouldn't others hear it too?

✓ **Listening to music:** Distract yourself with music, podcasts, or audiobooks.

✓ **Humming or singing:** Hum, sing or whistle a song. Doing so activates the areas of the brain responsible for processing sound. This helps the brain to fill the auditory space with real, intended sounds, which can reduce the intensity of hearing voices.

✓ **Mouth exercises:** Open your mouth wide and then close it again. This movement stimulates sensory feedback from the mouth and jaw, which can "ground" the brain and also activate your brain in a way that distracts from or competes with the auditory hallucinations, making them less noticeable.

✓ **Relaxation exercises:** Find suggestions for relaxation exercises on the worksheet "Positive Activities".

✓ **STOP:** Say "Stop" out loud. If it's not possible to say it out loud, then think it, and visualise a stop sign.

✓ **Search game:** Look around you and identify as quickly as possible five things that are red, five things that are blue, five things that are yellow.

✓ **Count:** Count backwards from 100.

✓ **Read aloud:** Read a passage of a text out loud to engage your focus.

✓ **Naming:** Point to an object in the room and name it out loud, continuing until everything in the room is named.

✓ **Stand against a wall:** So you can be sure that no one can stand behind you and talk to you.

✓ **Chasing away:** Tell the voices you don't want to talk to them. Send them away. You can get angry and shout at the voices to shut up.

✓ **Stop listening:** Cover your ears.

✓ **Distraction:** Do something to distract yourself, such as something from the list of positive activities. `

Fig. 5.7 (continued)

✓ **Ground yourself:** Hearing voices can make you feel like you are drifting away. You can counteract this feeling by actively seeking contact with the here and now. The easiest way to do this is to touch a wall or a fixed, stable object such as a table. Another way is to press your feet into the floor as hard as you can.

✓ **See through the voices:** Keep a log or diary to record when the voices occur, in what form, how strong they are, and under what circumstances. This can help you to recognise patterns in your voices and make them more predictable for you.

✓ **What do the voices want to tell you?** In psychology we assume that every symptom represents a need that is not being met sufficiently at the moment. Think about what needs the voices might be pointing to. What might they be trying to tell you?

✓ **Ignore them:** Sometimes, despite trying all of the above, the voices may not go away. If this happens, the voices aren't real and they can't hurt you. Don't give them power over you. Always remember that you don't have to do what they say. Just do what you want. If the voices tell you that something bad will happen if you don't obey them, stop and ask yourself: how often has what they said actually come true?

Own Ideas:

✓ ...

✓ ...

✓ ...

Fig. 5.7 (continued)

Concentration Problems

We all have moments when we cannot concentrate. Sometimes our thoughts are too distracting, or we feel too tired to focus. There are also times when our ability to concentrate seems limited for other various reasons. However, it is important not to give up and to keep trying to concentrate. You can improve your concentration with regular practice. Here are some tips to try when you feel like you can't concentrate.

Tips for dealing with concentration difficulties:

- ✓ **Memory training:** Concentration can be improved with practice. The more you practise, the better you will be able to concentrate. Exercises from the worksheet "Positive Activities" can help improve your ability to concentrate.
- ✓ **Time to concentrate:** Create a daily schedule of your free time and set aside specific windows of time in your calendar for focused work. Focus and work during these times, then take a break.
- ✓ **Optimal time of day for concentration:** Everyone has different times when they're most focused. Find out when you can concentrate best during the day. Try to do the task that requires a lot of concentration at that time. For example, if you find that you're less receptive after 8pm, don't schedule your study session then.
- ✓ **Ideal workplace:** Find a quiet, distraction-free place where you can concentrate on your work. Important: Not everyone works well at home - some people find it easier to study in a library or a quiet café. Find out where you can concentrate best.
- ✓ **Support tools:** Find tools to help you focus. Sometimes quiet background music, a warm cup of tea or a light snack can help. Try to find out what works best for you to help you focus.
- ✓ **Only 10 minutes:** Sit down and try to focus on something for just ten minutes. After that, if you're focus fades, you can do something else.
- ✓ **Step by step:** Sometimes it helps to turn a large piece of work into many small pieces. Start with the first step. Instead of trying to read a whole chapter, start by reading a single page.
- ✓ **Start with the easiest:** Do the task that seems easiest to you first.
- ✓ **Short break**: Listen to your favourite song. After the song ends, give the task another try.
- ✓ **Fresh air:** A short walk outside can help clear your mind. Walk around the block and then try to focus again.
- ✓ **Relaxation exercises:** Sometimes we are just too distracted and can't focus at all. It can be helpful to take a few minutes to relax, for example by doing a relaxation exercise - and then return to the task with renewed attention.
- ✓ **Organise your thoughts:** May be you cannot concentrate because you have too much on your mind. Write down all your thoughts and try again afterwards.
- ✓ **Pause**: Sometimes, concentration just won't happen. If it just isn't working, take a break and try again after 30 minutes.

Fig. 5.7 (continued)

- ✓ **Daily self-care:** You won't be able to concentrate if you're hungry, thirsty, or tired. Take care of yourself and make sure your basic needs are met.
- ✓ **Energy balance:** On days when you find it hard to concentrate, don't overload yourself. It is important to use your energy wisely. Prioritise important tasks and leave non-urgent ones for later.
- ✓ **Reassess your expectations:** Emotional problems such as low mood can lead to severe concentration problems. It is normal not to be able to meet all your expectations at the moment. You would not expect to study for an exam if you were in bed with the flu. Try to adjust your expectations to your current state of mind.

Own Ideas:

- ✓ …
- ✓ …
- ✓ …

Fig. 5.7 (continued)

Thought Disturbances

Many young people report that they suddenly notice a deterioration in their ability to think. For example, they can only think very slowly and logical thinking is very difficult for them. Or they experience mental blocks. Others report difficulties finding words or that sentences are no longer understood. Short-term memory can suddenly become worse. Reading or learning can become more difficult.

However, you are not simply at the mercy of these thinking difficulties. With targeted training and practice, you can improve your thinking again. This so-called cognitive training doesn't have to be strenuous. There are several strategies that you can try.

Tips for dealing with thinking difficulties

- ✓ **Memory training:** Concentration can be improved with practice. The more you practise, the better you will be able to concentrate. Exercises from the worksheet "Positive Activities" can help improve your ability to concentrate.
- ✓ **Spaghetti:** Tense all your muscles for a moment, then release them. This simple technique can help you refocus.
- ✓ **Relaxation exercises:** Sometimes we just get too distracted and can't stay focused. It can be helpful to take a few minutes to relax, for example by doing a relaxation exercise. Then return to the task with renewed attention.
- ✓ **Step by step:** Sometimes it helps to turn a large piece of work into many small pieces. Start with the first step. Instead of trying to read a whole chapter, start by reading a single page.
- ✓ **Start with the easiest:** Do the task that seems easiest to you first.
- ✓ **Fresh air:** A short walk outside can help clear your mind. Walk around the block and then try to focus again.
- ✓ **Organise your thoughts:** May be you cannot concentrate because you have too much on your mind. Write down all your thoughts and try again afterwards.
- ✓ **Short break**: If you feel mentally blocked, can't study, or have too many thoughts running through your head, try taking a short break from whatever you are doing. Listen to your favourite song, take a deep breath of fresh air, or drink a glass of water.

Own Ideas

- ✓ ...
- ✓ ...
- ✓ ...

Fig. 5.7 (continued)

Delusion

A delusion is when someone judges reality in a completely different way to everyone else. These thoughts or beliefs are often unusual and disconnected from the experiences of other people. They are frequently held despite evidence to the contrary.
Examples include

- Feeling special, superior to others, or believing you have special powers.
- A feeling of being watched or of being followed,
- A belief that you are in danger, or that there is some kind of conspiracy going on.
- The idea that your thoughts can be controlled from the outside, so that they can be removed, stolen, or inserted by others.
- Believing that your thoughts can be read or heard by others.

Tips for dealing with paranoia:

✓ **Thoughts ≠ Facts:** Just because you think something doesn't mean that it's necessarily true. Sometimes thoughts are wrong or just don't make sense. You don't always have to believe them. Remember that thoughts can be incorrect, and we're all wrong at times.

✓ **Stop thinking:** When strange or upsetting thoughts occur, say "stop" out loud or picture a stop sign in your mind to interrupt these thoughts.

✓ **Facts, not assumptions:** When you think about certain situations and they seem odd to you, check the facts. What happened and when did it happen? What are the objective facts of the situation that you can be sure of and that everyone else can agree on? Then stick to those facts and don't try to speculate about how or why something happened.

✓ **Double-check how likely it is:** How likely is it that your beliefs are correct? Are there other possibilities or explanations? Try to think about these possible explanations and how likely they are to be true.

✓ **Collect counter-evidence:** Is there any counter-evidence that contradicts your theories? Actively look for evidence that contradicts your theories. This can help to balance your perspective.

✓ **Question the connection:** Don't look for connections between two independent events. Coincidences happen, but that doesn't mean there's a meaningful connection.

✓ **Remain sceptical:** Question unusual thoughts and be sceptical about new ones. Challenge your thoughts, especially odd ones, with caution and curiosity.

✓ **Ask about it:** Ask your friends, family, or someone you trust about your thoughts. Share them with that person. If you suspect someone is plotting against you, talk to them about your concerns. Open communication can help clear up misunderstandings.

Fig. 5.7 (continued)

✓ **Question your automatic thoughts:** Many thoughts happen so quickly that we are not even consciously aware of them. These thought patterns are called automatic thoughts, and each of us has automatic thought patterns. This makes sense in everyday life because we would be overwhelmed if we had to actively think about every single thing all the time. But automatic thoughts can also lead to wrong conclusions. Try to work with your therapist to find out which automatic thought patterns you are prone to. Together you can look for strategies to help you recognise and challenge these thoughts.

✓ **Distraction:** Engage in activities that distract you from intrusive thoughts, such as something from the list of positive activities.

Own ideas:

✓ …

✓ …

✓ …

Fig. 5.7 (continued)

Anxiety

When we feel threatened, we react with fear. Fear is a natural biological reaction and all life forms have this instinct. It is an automatic response that prepares the body to fight or flight in response to perceived threats. Within seconds and without conscious awareness, the physical reaction to fear mobilises all of the body's resources. Common physical symptoms include a racing heart, trembling, dizziness or shortness of breath.

It is important to remind yourself that this feeling of fear or panic is temporary and will pass on its own. Remember that you are not powerless against anxiety. There are several coping skills you can learn to use in these situations.

Tips for dealing with anxiety:

- ✓ **Refocus:** When you feel anxious, accept its presence, then let it go and concentrate on what you wanted to do. Take three deep breaths, try to relax your body, smile and say to yourself: "Hello fear. I've noticed you're here. But now I'm going to leave".
- ✓ **Relaxation exercises:** Try to relax. Anxiety will decrease. See the worksheet "Positive Activities" for relaxation techniques to help in stressful moments.
- ✓ **Spaghetti:** Tense all your muscles at the same time, hold for a moment, and then release them all.
- ✓ **Breathing techniques:** In moments of anxiety, we tend to breathe faster. Try to slow down your breathing, breathing in and out slowly.
- ✓ **Slow steps:** Slowly take three steps forward and then backwards.
- ✓ **Count:** Count backwards from 100.
- ✓ **Read out loud:** Read a passage of text out loud.
- ✓ **Have a drink:** Drink a glass of water
- ✓ **Close your eyes:** Close your eyes, take a deep breath, and then open your eyes again.
- ✓ **Jump:** Jump up and down on your right leg five times and then on your left leg five times.
- ✓ **Name things:** Ground yourself by naming five things you see, four things you can hear and three things you can feel.
- ✓ **Hum a song.** Humming can slow down the heartbeat, promote deep breathing, and create calming vibrations in the body.
- ✓ **Assess your posture:** Face your fear with an upright, open, and strong posture. Keep your back straight, shoulders down, chest out, stomach in, and head up.
- ✓ **Ground yourself**: Actively seek contact with the here and now. The easiest way to do this is to touch a wall or a fixed, stable object such as a table. Another option is to press your feet against the floor as hard as you can.
- ✓ **Fear is just a feeling:** Just because you're scared doesn't mean there's a real danger. Remind yourself that fear is just a feeling.
- ✓ **Reality check:** Analyse and question your fears. Is your fear justified? Is there really a danger right now? And even if there is danger, is your level of fear justified? Do you really need to be so afraid?
- ✓ **Do the opposite.** Don't give your anxiety any power. It is not a good counsellor. Instead, try to do the opposite of what your fear tells you to do.

Fig. 5.7 (continued)

- ✓ **The fear will pass:** Like all emotions, fear is temporary. There is no feeling that lasts forever. Just as we are not always happy, it is impossible to be afraid all the time. Try to remind yourself that your anxiety is temporary and will pass.

Own Ideas:

- ✓ …
- ✓ …
- ✓ …

Fig. 5.7 (continued)

Sleeping Problems

Regular and sufficient sleep is very important for general wellbeing. However, during stressful times, many people struggle to fall asleep, wake up frequently during the night, or find it difficult to go back to sleep.

There are several strategies you can try to improve the quality of your sleep.

- ✓ **Regular bedtimes:** Try to keep to a regular bedtime if possible.
- ✓ **Sleep only at night:** Avoid naps during the day, even if you feel tired.
- ✓ **Your bed is a quiet area:** You should only use your bed for sleeping. Not as a place to study, eat, watch movies, surf the web, etc.
- ✓ **Bedtime routines:** Think about a bedtime ritual, such as taking a warm bath, drinking a cup of tea, or listening to calming music.
- ✓ **Mobile device ban:** Don't take your mobile phone to bed.
- ✓ **Electric-free zone:** No electronic devices in the bedroom.
- ✓ **Avoid caffeine:** Excessive consumption of caffeine (in coffee, iced tea, energy drinks, etc.) can lead to sleep problems. Moderate consumption of caffeine-containing substances is a prerequisite for good sleep quality, especially in the second half of the day, as these substances have a long duration of action. Try not to drink coffee, energy drinks, or other stimulating drinks after 4 pm.
- ✓ **Check the temperature:** Make sure that the temperature in your room is not too hot or too cold.
- ✓ **Dark room:** Make sure it is dark enough.
- ✓ **Avoid excitement:** Before going to bed, try to avoid activities that could agitate or excite you, such as excessive exercise or watching horror films.
- ✓ **Go offline**: Messages (or not messages...) on social media can unnecessarily upset you. An hour or two before going to bed, try turning off your phone or putting it away.
- ✓ **Write down your thoughts**: Ruminating at night can make it difficult to fall asleep and is not helpful. Especially before we fall asleep, we make many problems seem more difficult than they really are. Things look different in the light of day. Put a pad next to your bed where you can write down your thoughts and review them the next day.
- ✓ **Don't look at the time:** Don't look at the time at night, it will only make you worry more.
- ✓ **Don't toss and turn in bed:** If you can't sleep at night, get up and do some quiet activity.
- ✓ **Warm or cold washcloth:** If you can't sleep, placing a warm or cold washcloth on your forehead may help. This can calm you down and help you focus on the here and now if you are too preoccupied with difficult thoughts. Alternatively, you can use a warm bedtime bottle.
- ✓ **Sleeping mask:** Using a sleeping mask can contribute to better sleep. Sleeping masks shield the eyes from external light sources. Another advantage is that a sleep mask

Fig. 5.7 (continued)

automatically causes the closing of the eyelids, which helps with general physical relaxation. Our body has learned to sleep when the eyelids remain closed.

✓ **Relaxation exercises:** If you have sleep problems, relaxation exercises can be helpful. You can find suggestions in the list of positive activities.

✓ **For once, you can do without it:** Even if you can't fall asleep, it's not a disaster. Although regular sleep is important for recovery, our bodies can cope with little or no sleep for a night. You can still function almost normally the next day, even if you are tired. Remember that even if you don't sleep, your body will rest if you lie still and relaxed in bed.

Own Ideas:

✓ ...

✓ ...

✓ ...

Fig. 5.7 (continued)

Substance Use

Drugs can provide temporary relief by calming you down, helping you to forget your problems or improving your mood. However, drugs can also make symptoms such as difficulty concentrating, hallucinations, paranoia, or depression worse. In some cases, drugs can even cause psychosis. It is therefore important that you use other strategies to improve your mood. These alternative strategies may not have the immediate effects of drugs, but they are much more helpful in the long term.

List the pros and cons of drug use with your therapist.

Substance Use

	Advantages	Disadvantages
short-term:		
long-term:		

Fig. 5.7 (continued)

Tips for addressing substance problems:

- ✓ **List of pros and cons:** Create a list of advantages and disadvantages of drugs.
- ✓ **Save the money**: Save the money you would normally spend on drugs and use it for something you've wanted for a long time.
- ✓ **Distraction:** Do something that distracts you, such as something from the list of positive activities.
- ✓ **Relaxation exercises:** Try to calm yourself with relaxation exercises. Check the list of positive activities for examples.
- ✓ **Educate yourself:** Research and read about the negative side effects of drug use online.
- ✓ **Confront the consequences:** Search the internet for before and after pictures of people who have used drugs.
- ✓ **Give up your old habits:** Change the routines that are linked to substance use into new ones. This might also include reflecting about your circle of friends.
- ✓ **Slow reduction:** Reduce your consumption slowly. Every small reduction is a step in the right direction and a success.

Own Ideas:

- ✓ …
- ✓ …
- ✓ …

Fig. 5.7 (continued)

Mood Protocol

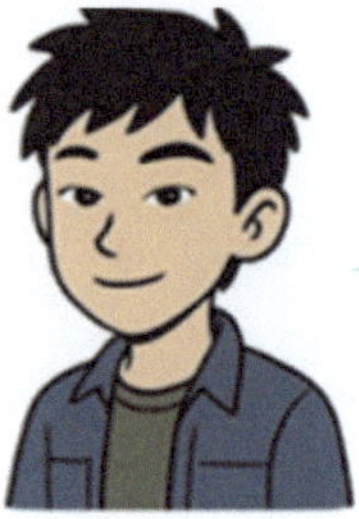

Every day, in the morning, at lunchtime, in the evening, and before you go to sleep, make a note of your mood. Rate your mood from 0 to 10.
0= I feel extremely bad
10= I feel extremely well

—— 2 —— 4 —— 6 —— 8 —— 10

	Morning	Noon	Evening	Night
Monday				
Tuesday				
Wednesday				
Thursday				
Friday				
Saturday				
Sunday				

Fig. 5.7 (continued)

Mood Protocol

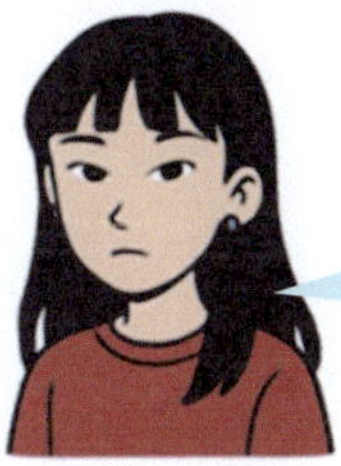

Every day, in the morning, at lunchtime, in the evening, and before you go to sleep, make a note of your mood. Red means you are feeling extremely bad. Green means you are feeling particularly good. Yellow means your mood is in the middle range.

	Morning	Noon	Evening	Night
Monday	☐ ☐ ☐	☐ ☐ ☐	☐ ☐ ☐	☐ ☐ ☐
Tuesday	☐ ☐ ☐	☐ ☐ ☐	☐ ☐ ☐	☐ ☐ ☐
Wednesday	☐ ☐ ☐	☐ ☐ ☐	☐ ☐ ☐	☐ ☐ ☐
Thursday	☐ ☐ ☐	☐ ☐ ☐	☐ ☐ ☐	☐ ☐ ☐
Friday	☐ ☐ ☐	☐ ☐ ☐	☐ ☐ ☐	☐ ☐ ☐
Saturday	☐ ☐ ☐	☐ ☐ ☐	☐ ☐ ☐	☐ ☐ ☐
Sunday	☐ ☐ ☐	☐ ☐ ☐	☐ ☐ ☐	☐ ☐ ☐

Fig. 5.7 (continued)

Mood Protocol

Assess your mood every day and record it in the journal. If your mood is in the green zone, you are doing well and not experiencing extreme moods. In the red area, you can describe your mood highs and lows.

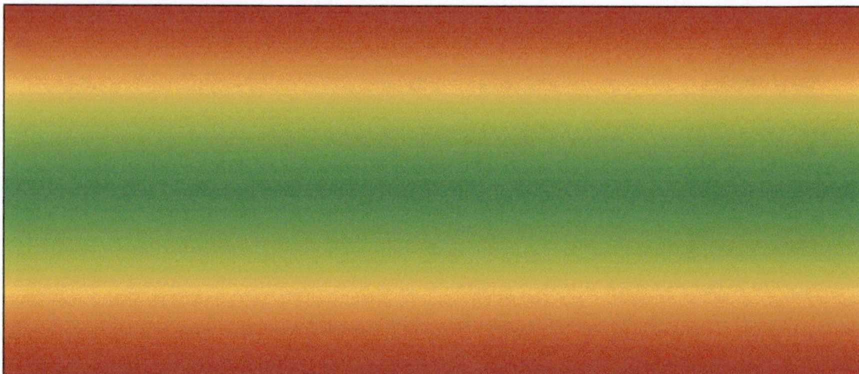

Monday	Tuesday	Wednesday	Thursday	Friday	Saturday	Sunday

Fig. 5.7 (continued)

Protocol of Positive Activities

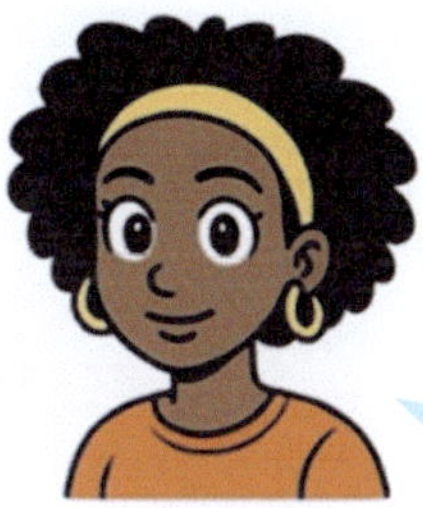

How we feel is closely linked to what we do. Activities that we enjoy automatically make us feel better. It is important to set aside time at least once a day to do something just for yourself. Try to choose at least one suggestion from the list of positive activities every day.

Rate your mood before and after doing the activity from 0 -10:

0= I feel extremely bad

10= I am doing extremely well

—— 2 —— 4 —— 6 —— 8 —— 10

	Monday	Tuesday	Wednesday	Thursday
activity				
Mood before/ after	/	/	/	/

	Friday	Saturday	Sunday
Activity			
Mood before / after	/	/	/

Fig. 5.7 (continued)

Protocol of positive activities

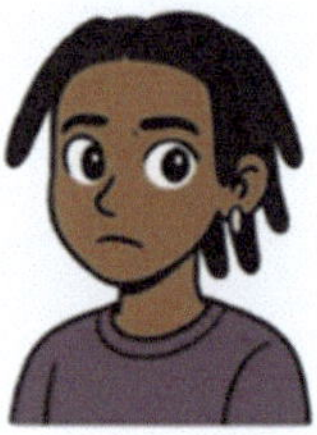

How we feel is closely linked to what we do. Activities that we enjoy automatically make us feel better. It is important to set aside time at least once a day to do something just for yourself. Try to choose at least one suggestion from the list of positive activities every day.

Assess your mood before and after you do the activity.

	Monday	Tuesday	Wednesday	Thursday
Activity				
Mood before / after	□□□/□□□	□□□/□□□	□□□/□□□	□□□/□□□

	Friday	Saturday	Sunday
Activity			
Mood before / after	□□□/ □□□	□□□/□□□	□□□/ □□□

Fig. 5.7 (continued)

Symptom Protocol

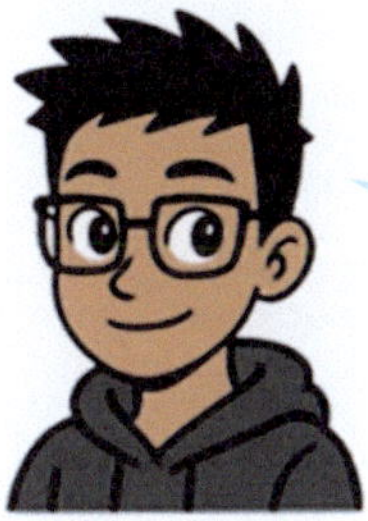

Make a list of your most common symptoms and observe how often they occur over the course of a week.

Symptom	Monday	Tuesday	Wednesday	Thursday	Friday	Saturday	Sunday

Fig. 5.7 (continued)

Dealing with my symptoms

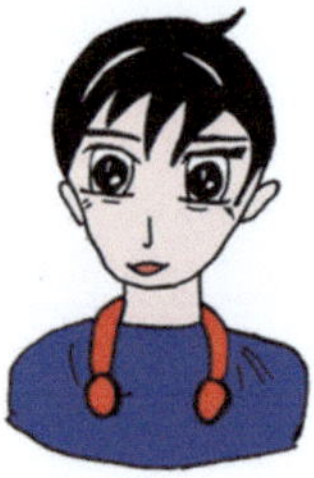

Note the situation and rate the severity of the symptom on a scale (1 = very mild to 10 = worse than ever). Choose a coping strategy from the list of tips and try it out. If the first strategy doesn't work, try another one. Keep experimenting until you find something that works. Don't give up, it may take time to discover what really helps. Once you've used a coping strategy, note how the intensity of the symptom changes (0 = no longer present, 1 = very mild, 10 = as strong as ever).

Symptom	Situation	Intensity (1-10)	Coping strategy 1	Coping strategy 2	Intensity (1-10)

Fig. 5.7 (continued)

Further Reading

Addington J, Francey S, Morrison AP, editors. Working with people at high risk of developing psychosis: a treatment handbook. Wiley; 2006.

Beaulieu D, Hoff H. Impact techniques for therapists. Routledge; 2013.

Catalan A, De Pablo GS, Aymerich C, Damiani S, Sordi V, Radua J, et al. Neurocognitive functioning in individuals at clinical high risk for psychosis: a systematic review and meta-analysis. JAMA Psychiatry. 2021;78(8):859–67.

Fusar-Poli P, Deste G, Smieskova R, Barlati S, Yung AR, Howes O, et al. Cognitive functioning in prodromal psychosis: a meta-analysis. Arch Gen Psychiatry. 2012;69(6):562–71.

Gleeson JF, McGorry PD, editors. Psychological interventions in early psychosis: a treatment handbook. Wiley; 2004.

Green MF, Kern RS, Heaton RK. Longitudinal studies of cognition and functional outcome in schizophrenia: implications for MATRICS. Schizophr Res. 2004;72(1):41–51.

Hedges EP, See C, Si S, McGuire P, Dickson H, Kempton MJ. Meta-analysis of longitudinal neurocognitive performance in people at clinical high-risk for psychosis. Psychol Med. 2022;52(11):2009–16.

Yung AR, Cotter J, McGorry PD. Youth mental health: approaches to emerging mental ill-Health in young people. Routledge; 2020.

Hypothetical Reasoning

6

Hypothetical reasoning is an important part of any psychological therapy with adolescents meeting CHR criteria, as it helps identify and challenge unfavorable thought patterns and paranoid causal chains. Unlike psychotic patients, patients with CHR symptoms are usually still able to engage in these processes and question their delusional thoughts. Nevertheless, adolescents with CHR symptoms often find it difficult to modify unfavorable thought patterns or to recognize paranoid or delusional thoughts as such. There are several reasons for this. Many adolescents meeting CHR criteria tend toward cognitive distortions, such as jumping to conclusions, finding causal links where they are not, or focusing only on arguments that confirm already-held hypotheses. Patients may also refuse to consider alternative points of view because they reveal a painful reality. All of these factors increase the importance for therapists to address the potential benefits of unfavorable thinking patterns for patients.

6.1 How Do Our Thought Patterns Develop?

Our way of thinking depends on various factors. For example, it is influenced by experiences as well as cultural norms and values. As adolescents' attitudes and beliefs are generally still quite fluid, a major challenge during adolescence is to create a personal value system. This requires a critical examination of previous family and cultural values at a time when peer groups become increasingly influential. Adolescents meeting CHR criteria are often particularly insecure about their previous beliefs, which increases the tendency toward one-sided perceptions.

Supplementary Information The online version contains supplementary material available at https://doi.org/10.1007/978-3-032-10341-3_6. The videos can be accessed individually by clicking the DOI link in the accompanying figure caption or by scanning this link with the SN More Media App.

N. Traber-Walker, M. Franscini, *Adolescents at Clinical High Risk for Psychosis*,
https://doi.org/10.1007/978-3-032-10341-3_6

Our current mood also plays an important role in how we perceive certain situations. A large proportion of patients with CHR symptoms suffer from mood swings, which are reflected in the way they think. During depressive phases, they tend to see themselves and the world very negatively, whereas during times of elevated mood, they are more confident and tend to make self-esteem-boosting attributions.

Therapy involves not only identifying patients' dysfunctional cognitions but also understanding why they are more susceptible to certain thought patterns than others. A non-judgmental attitude is therefore essential.

Case Example: Lucy

Toward the end of primary school, Lucy experienced a brief period of bullying from her classmates. She doesn't remember exactly how it started, but it was mainly one girl who suddenly targeted Lucy with hurtful comments. The girl accused Lucy of being vain and arrogant, even calling her a "prima ballerina." Other classmates joined in, laughing at the cruel remarks, and Lucy felt increasingly isolated. After a five-week period that was very distressing for Lucy, the summer holidays provided a temporary reprieve in which Lucy had no contact with her classmates.

When school started again, it was as though everything that had occurred previously had been forgotten. No one was mean to Lucy, and her friends acted as if nothing had changed. However, Lucy remembers that time as very painful and prefers not to think about it. Fortunately, nothing like that has ever happened again. Lucy has always been popular and has many friends. However, she has become very sensitive and tends to take others' comments personally. She has a deep-seated fear that people will suddenly turn against her again, making her more susceptible to distrust and paranoid thoughts about her peers.

Case Example: Michael

Michael's school career was not without its challenges. In particular, his attention deficit disorder made it difficult for him to get the grades he needed. In primary school, he often clashed with teachers who perceived him as lazy or even stupid. Thanks to treatment with methylphenidate, his academic situation improved toward the end of primary school. Despite this progress, Michael maintains a certain distrust of teachers. He is quick to feel unfairly judged by them. He is also sensitive to poor grades or learning difficulties. As a result of his CHR symptoms, Michael is currently experiencing a decline in cognitive functioning, which is causing him considerable concern and anxiety.

6.2 Typical Errors in Reasoning

A majority of adolescents meeting CHR criteria are prone to cognitive distortions that contribute to the continuation and reinforcement of symptoms. For example, patients with paranoid thoughts often recall the attributions that support their paranoid ideas more quickly, whereas alternative explanatory models are rarely considered. Paranoid or depressive beliefs are thus supported and maintained, regardless of actual experience or counter-arguments. Some of the typical cognitive distortions of patients with CHR symptoms are described in the following.

Jumping to Conclusions

Jumping to conclusions refers to making a quick judgment about a situation or person based on a first impression, without considering that there may not be enough information to make an accurate or reliable assessment. Research has shown that people with psychotic disorders tend to use significantly less information when forming an opinion than do healthy people. This cognitive pattern is also seen in patients with CHR symptoms. Jumping to conclusions can contribute to the development of delusional thoughts by encouraging rushed and often inaccurate reasoning. In therapy, it is therefore important to guide patients to consider evidence and context carefully before drawing conclusions, rather than relying on immediate assumptions.

Example

Lucy always feels that one of her classmates has something against her, so much so that she is even plotting against Lucy. One Monday morning, Lucy arrives at school an hour late because of a doctor's appointment. Lucy doesn't know that this classmate made an announcement before class, stating she was having a birthday party and inviting everyone in the class. The announcement was also shared on the class WhatsApp group, but Lucy hasn't seen it yet. During break, the whole class is talking about the party. Lucy thinks: "I knew it. She's completely against me. Now she's having a party that everyone knows about because everyone is invited—except for me." Lucy feels so sad and excluded that she immediately deletes the class chat on her mobile phone. She never reads the message that she, too, was invited.

All-or-Nothing Thinking

All-or-nothing thinking is also known as black-and-white thinking or polarized thinking. This type of thinking involves looking at things in absolute terms: Situations are always black or white, all or nothing, good or bad, or success or failure. There is no gradient. Many adolescents tend to take an extreme view of things. Depressive and delusional symptoms often lead patients to become even more trapped in this way of thinking.

Example

Michael has an important exam tomorrow. He thinks: If I do badly in this exam, I won't have to continue my apprenticeship.

Overgeneralization

Overgeneralization occurs when people draw broad conclusions from a single event or a series of coincidences. Having experienced an event in a certain way, they assume that future events will happen in the same way. This leads to the creation of a general rule based on a single negative experience. Adolescents in particular tend to make such sweeping generalizations, often using words such as "never" or "always," thereby reinforcing rigid beliefs.

> **Example**
> A boy Lucy likes asks her friend Tina to dance at a party. Lucy is then convinced: "All the boys like Tina more than they like me. Nobody ever wants to dance with me."

Internal or External Causal Attribution

Internal and external attribution styles refer to how people explain the causes of events or behaviors by attributing them to either internal (within themselves) or external (outside themselves) factors. People with an internal attribution style tend to see the origin of an event in their own person and behavior. In contrast, people with an external attribution style tend to externalize the cause, i.e., attributing it to other people or external circumstances rather than to themselves. Both exclusively internal and exclusively external causal attributions are common in adolescents with CHR symptoms. Patients with delusions often tend to externalize the causes of ambiguous events. Internal attribution styles, on the other hand, are common in patients with depressive symptoms or guilt-related beliefs. The way in which an event is justified has a major influence on our state of mind. Patients with an external attribution style often feel helpless and at the mercy of the world because external factors cannot be influenced. Internal causal attributions, on the other hand, lead to excessive responsibility, feelings of guilt, or a negative self-image.

> **Example**
> Michael is well-prepared for his math exam. He has studied on his own and with a tutor. Since Michael has solved all the exercises correctly, he believes that he understands the material and goes into the exam with confidence. During the exam, however, the tasks are much more difficult than the exercises. Michael does not understand several tasks and receives an unsatisfactory grade.

Example

External attribution

Michael thinks: I can prepare and study as much as I want. In the end, this math teacher always gives such difficult exams, so I will fail regardless. It's no use. Next time I won't study at all.

Internal attribution

Michael thinks: No matter how much I study, I won't be able to succeed in the end. I'm just too stupid. I'll never manage this apprenticeship regardless of how hard I try.

Discounting the Positive

Discounting the positive is a cognitive distortion that involves ignoring or invalidating good things that have happened. The positive experiences are not valued equally or are dismissed as exceptions. This leads to the maintenance of negative beliefs, even when the patient has numerous countervailing experiences.

Example

Lucy performs the new choreography in her dance group so well that the teacher praises her for it. In the next round or rehearsal, Lucy takes a step to the right instead of the left, bumping into a fellow dancer. In the final round, however, Lucy performs everything correctly. When Lucy goes home after class, she feels completely frustrated. She is so embarrassed that she danced in the wrong direction. She has completely forgotten about the teacher's praise.

Emotional Reasoning

Emotional reasoning is a way of judging oneself or circumstances based on emotions only. This type of reasoning assumes that because a negative emotion is experienced, it must be an accurate reflection of reality. The presence of this emotion is taken as confirmation of a particular assumption, even though there is no objective evidence to support this assumption.

Example

Michael feels uneasy when he walks home late at night. It is dark, and he feels afraid. He thinks: Something is wrong here. I'm scared, so someone must be following me; otherwise, I wouldn't be scared.

Personalization

This is the tendency to feel responsible for a negative event regardless of the direct level of involvement. This thought pattern frequently occurs in patients with relationship ideation.

> **Example**
> Lucy's younger sister sprains her ankle during a trial class at Lucy's dance school. Lucy thinks: It's my fault because I told my sister about the class. If I hadn't, she wouldn't have gone, and she wouldn't have sprained her ankle.

Catastrophizing

This is the tendency to assume the worst possible outcome. The tendency to overdramatize is considered typical of adolescents. In adolescents with CHR symptoms, catastrophizing is often more pronounced than in their peers, as many CHR symptoms are conducive to this type of thinking. For example, patients who hear voices often report that these voices predict such catastrophes.

> **Example**
> Michael misses the bus in the morning and will be late for work. He thinks: "My boss is going to be very angry. He might even fire me." Michael decides not to go to work. Instead, he goes home and calls in sick.

Selective Perception

Selective perception is a cognitive bias in which individuals focus on certain aspects of a situation or experience while ignoring or downplaying other relevant information. This bias leads them to interpret events in a way that is consistent with their pre-existing beliefs, emotions, or expectations, rather than considering a more balanced or objective perspective. In particular, patients with paranoid symptoms look for evidence in everyday life that supports their paranoid thoughts. Evidence to the contrary is ignored. Selective perception distorts reality by narrowing the patient's focus, leading them to draw conclusions based on incomplete or distorted information. As a result, negative thought patterns such as feelings of inadequacy, mistrust, or hopelessness may be reinforced.

> **Example**
> Lucy gets a haircut. After the appointment, she feels very insecure about it and thinks that her head looks huge with the new hairstyle. The next day, however, she receives many compliments from her classmates about her new haircut. Even her secret crush tells Lucy that the shorter hair looks good on her. In the evening after school, Lucy bumps into an old primary school friend whom she hasn't seen in over a year. She says nothing about Lucy's hair. Afterward, Lucy is convinced: "My new haircut doesn't look good. My head looks so big now."

In our clinical experience, it is not helpful for the therapist to explain to the patient the nature of their dysfunctional thought patterns. Particularly with paranoid patients, this can reinforce the impression that the therapist is "against them." In contrast, general psychoeducation using case examples of typical cognitive distortions is recommended. Patients can be given the worksheet "Typical Cognitive Distortions." It illustrates the cognitive distortions mentioned here with examples from Lucy and Michael. As a first step, patients can take a moment to think about which of these cognitive distortions they recognize in themselves.

6.3 Hypothetical Reasoning in Therapy

A key component of therapy is helping patients reframe dysfunctional thought patterns that negatively affect their well-being. The therapist may use Socratic questioning to guide the patient through this process. This method is non-directive and does not aim to establish right or wrong answers. Instead, it is a gradual and collaborative exercise where the patient learns to generate alternative hypotheses. The goal is not to assert a definitive truth but to explore the emotional and behavioral consequences of different hypotheses and assess their likelihood.

As mentioned earlier, for some patients, it may be easier not to start with their own personal experiences. Depending on the severity of their symptoms, these could be too overwhelming. The first two hypothetical thinking worksheets contain case studies of Lucy and Michael. These case studies serve as a first step in helping patients recognize the impact of unhelpful thinking patterns in everyday situations. Patients are encouraged to generate alternative hypotheses about the events in Lucy's or Michael's life, assess the emotions these might evoke, and evaluate the likelihood that the proposed explanations are accurate.

As patients become more comfortable with this approach, the technique of hypothetical thinking can be applied to their personal experiences. Patients can use a protocol to document challenging situations, which can then be analyzed during therapy.

The first step is for the patient to describe the situation objectively. They then write down their thoughts and assumptions: How did they interpret the situation? What feelings did this interpretation evoke? How did their interpretation affect their behavior? The worksheet "My Typical Thoughts and Beliefs" can help patients identify recurrent cognitive patterns. The therapist should lead a discussion about the advantages and disadvantages of these thoughts. After this exercise, the patient should be encouraged to develop alternative thought patterns and possible strategies for dealing with the situation. These can be recorded on the worksheet "Alternative Explanatory Models," similar to the examples with Lucy and Michael.

The next step is to instruct patients to develop different hypotheses about a particular event, focusing on finding evidence against their unfavorable interpretations. The final worksheet, 'Finding alternative explanations,' is designed for this purpose. This technique may be useful for reviewing past situations during therapy and then having patients apply it to future events as homework.

6.4 Worksheets

The following worksheets (Fig. 6.1) belong to this chapter and are available online for download in the context of the electronic chapter:

- Worksheet 32 "Hypothetical Reasoning"
- Worksheet 33 "Hypothetical Reasoning: Protocol of Your Own Example"
- Worksheet 34 "My Typical Thoughts and Beliefs"
- Worksheet 35 "Hypothetical Reasoning: Typical Thinking Errors"
- Worksheet 36 "Hypothetical Reasoning: Alternative Explanatory Models"
- Worksheet 37 "Hypothetical Reasoning: Find Alternative Explanations"

Hypothetical Reasoning

Each of us has certain thought patterns. We all interpret and evaluate certain events in our own way. The way we interpret certain events depends on many factors. For example, these might include experiences, beliefs, personality traits, and psychological impairments.

Example: Lucy has been invited to a friend's birthday party next week, but she is not really looking forward to the party. She hardly knows anyone other than the party host.

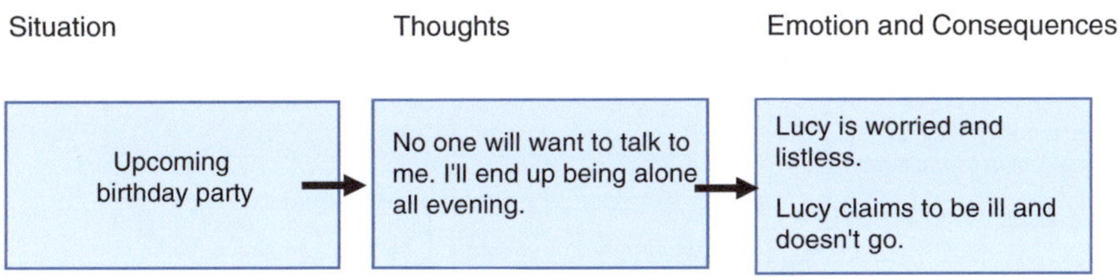

Hypothetical reasoning is about questioning and rethinking the way we see and perceive certain things.

Example: Lucy rethinks her situation, questioning her original thoughts.

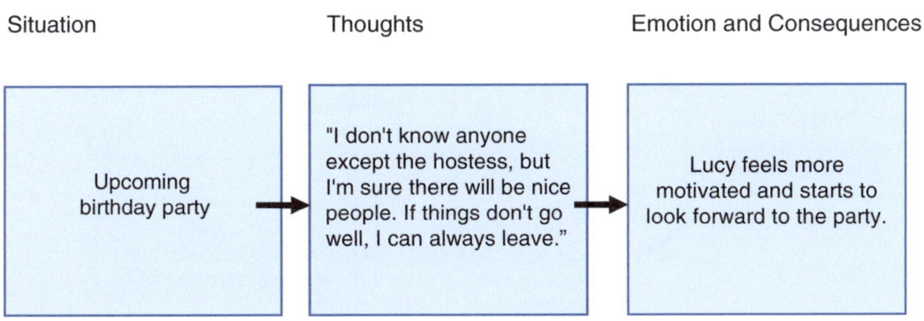

Fig. 6.1 Worksheet 32 to Worksheet 37

There are several explanations for most events. However, we often make the mistake of focusing our attention on only one possible explanation. This can make it difficult to deal with the situation. Especially when we're not feeling well, we tend to adopt certain negative perspectives and often interpret situations to our disadvantage.
Here are a few more examples:

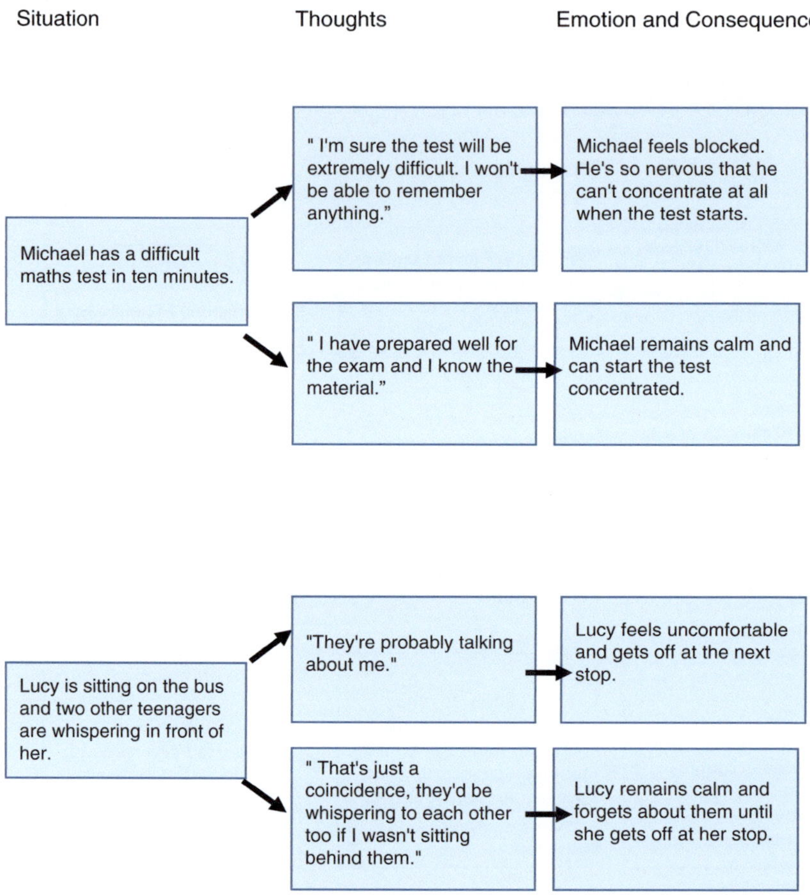

Fig. 6.1 (continued)

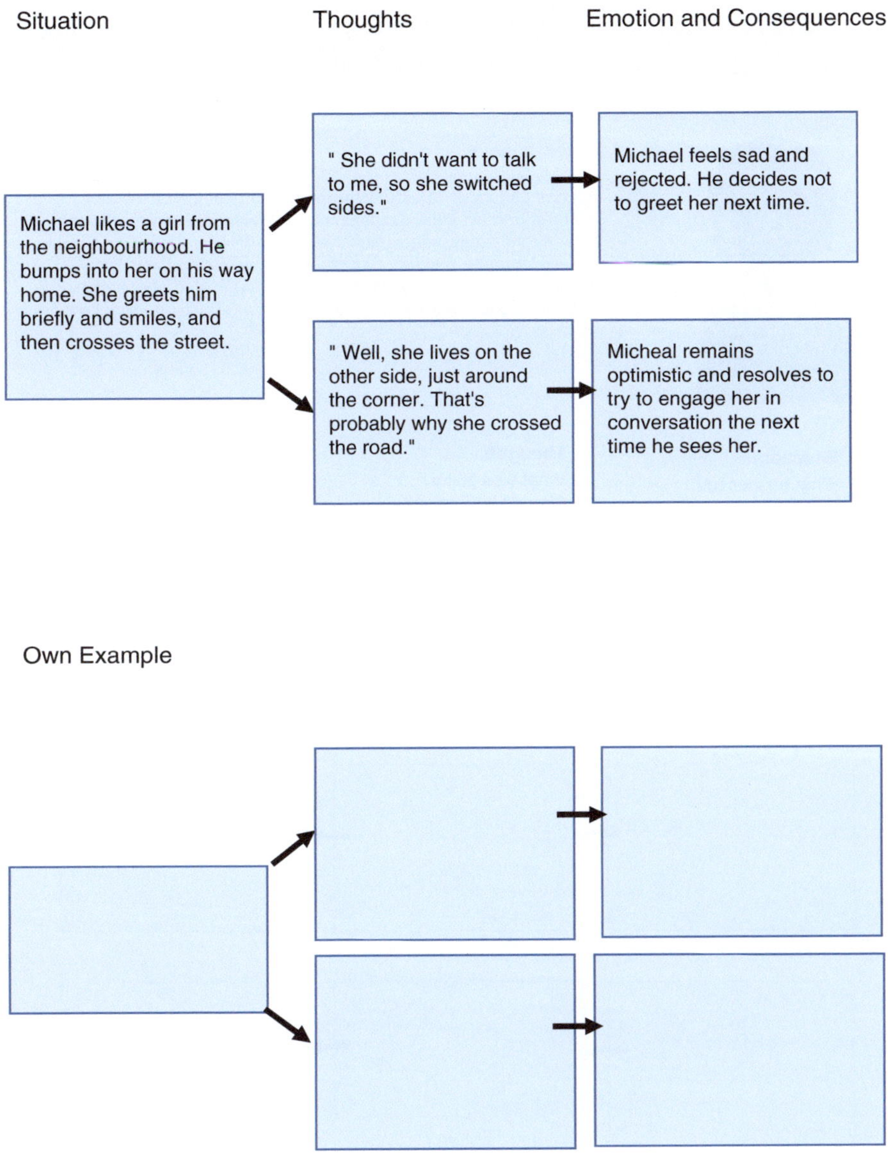

Fig. 6.1 (continued)

Hypothetical Reasoning: Protocol of Your Own Examples

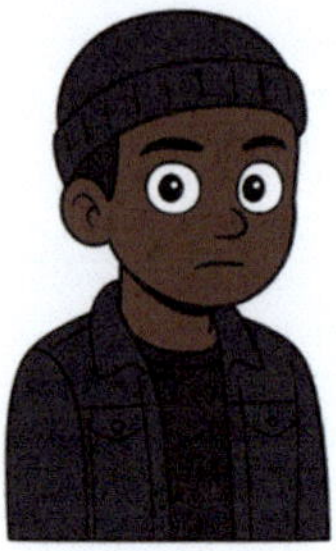

Each of us has certain thought patterns, meaning that we all interpret and evaluate events in our own way. The interpretation of an event in turn affects how we feel and how we behave. Until the next therapy session, record various events that you experience in your daily life. Note what thoughts you have along with these experiences how the thoughts affect your feelings and behaviour.

Situation:
What happened?

Thoughts:
What was going through your mind?

Consequences:
How did it make you feel?
How did you react?

Fig. 6.1 (continued)

My Typical Thoughts and Beliefs

My typical thoughts and beliefs	Advantages of these beliefs	Disadvantages of these beliefs	Possible alternatives for my thoughts and assumptions

Fig. 6.1 (continued)

Hypothetical Reasoning: Typical Thinking Errors

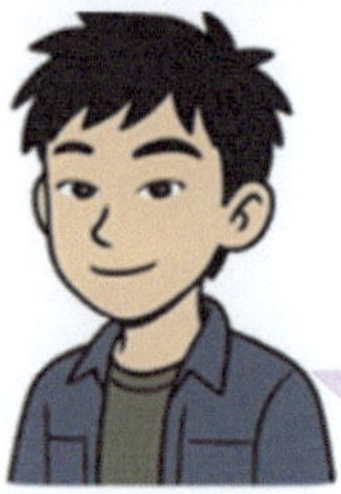

A large proportion of our thoughts occur so quickly that we are not even consciously aware of them. These thought patterns are called automatic thoughts, and everyone has them. This is useful in everyday life because we would be overwhelmed if we had to think about everything consciously all the time. However, automatic thoughts can also lead to thinking errors, which can negatively affect our mood and behaviour. Below are some of the most common thinking errors. Read the explanations and case studies, and then discuss with your therapist which of these thinking errors sound familiar to you.

Jumping to conclusions: This means that we immediately have an opinion on something even though we may not know everything yet. No consideration is given to the fact that we may still have too little information to make a reliable statement. Example:Lucy feels that one of her classmates has something against her or is even plotting against her. One Monday morning, Lucy arrives at school an hour late after a doctor's appointment. Lucy doesn't know that during the morning, while she was visiting the doctor, this classmate made an announcement, declaring she was having a birthday party and inviting everyone in the class to attend. The announcement was also shared on the class WhatsApp group, but Lucy hasn't seen it yet. During break, the whole class is talking about the party. Lucy thinks: "I knew it. She's trying to keep me out. Everyone is talking about her party because everyone is invited - except me". Lucy feels so sad and excluded that she immediately deletes the class chat on her mobile phone. She never reads the message that she was invited, too.

All or nothing principle: This is when we have an extreme view of things and think in black and white terms. Example: Michael has an important exam tomorrow. He thinks: If I do badly in this exam, I won't have to continue my apprenticeship.

Exaggerated generalizations: This is when we create a general principle from a single negative event. Example: A boy Lucy likes asks her friend Tina to dance at a party. Lucy is then convinced: "All the boys like Tina more than me. Nobody ever wants to dance with me."

Internal or external causal attribution: This means we attribute the cause of an ambiguous event to ourselves (internal factors), the behaviour of another person (external factors), or the situation (also external). The way we explain an event significantly impacts how we feel. When we attribute causes to external factors, we often feel helpless and at the mercy of circumstances. The factors seem beyond our control. When we attribute causes to internal factors, we can have feelings of responsibility, guilt, or a negative self-image.

Example: Michael has prepared very well for his maths exam. He has studied with his tutor and is confident that he understands the material. He has done all the exercises correctly and is optimistic about the exam. However, the questions in the exam are much more difficult than the exercises. Michael struggles to understand some of the questions and receives an unsatisfactory grade.

External attribution of causes:
Michael thinks: I can prepare and study as much as I want. In the end, this maths teacher always gives such difficult exams that I will still fail. It's no use, so next time I won't study at all.
Internal attribution of causes:

Fig. 6.1 (continued)

Michael thinks: No matter how much I study, in the end, I won't be able to do it. I'm just too stupid. I'll never manage this apprenticeship, no matter how hard I try.

Ignoring positive experiences: This is when we ignore positive experiences, even when many exist, allowing negative beliefs to persist. When we experience good things or are successful at something, it is not considered as important as the negative things or it is dismissed as an exception. Example: Lucy performs a new choreography in her dance group so well that the teacher praises her for it. In the next round, Lucy takes a step to the right instead of the left, bumping into a fellow dancer. In the final round of choreography, however, everything works as it should. When Lucy goes home after class, she feels completely frustrated. She is so embarrassed that she danced in the wrong direction, and she has completely forgotten about the teacher's praise.

Emotional reasoning: This means that a final opinion is formed on the basis of a single feeling. The presence of this feeling is taken as confirmation of a particular assumption, even though there are no other clues to support it. Example: Michael feels uneasy when he walks home late at night. It is dark and he feels afraid. He thinks: Something is wrong here. I'm scared, so someone must be following me, otherwise I wouldn't be scared.

Personalization: This refers to our tendency to feel responsible for a negative event even though we had nothing to do with it. Example: Lucy's younger sister sprains her ankle during a trial class at Lucy's dance school. Lucy thinks: It's my fault because I told my sister about the class. If I hadn't, she wouldn't have gone, and she wouldn't have sprained her ankle.

Catastrophising: This means we tend to assume the worst possible outcome in a situation. Example: Michael misses the bus in the morning and will be late for work. He thinks: "My boss is going to be very angry. He might even fire me." Michael decides not to go to work. Instead, he goes home and calls in sick.

Selective perception: This is when we only pay attention to factors and events that support our assumptions. Evidence to the contrary is ignored. Example:Lucy gets her hair cut. She feels insecure about how it looks and thinks the new style makes her head look huge. The next day, however, she receives many compliments about the new haircut from her classmates. Even her secret crush tells Lucy that the shorter hair looks good on her. After school, Lucy bumps into an old primary school friend whom she hasn't seen in over a year. The girl says nothing about Lucy's hair. Afterwards, Lucy is convinced: "My new haircut doesn't look good, my head looks so big now".

Fig. 6.1 (continued)

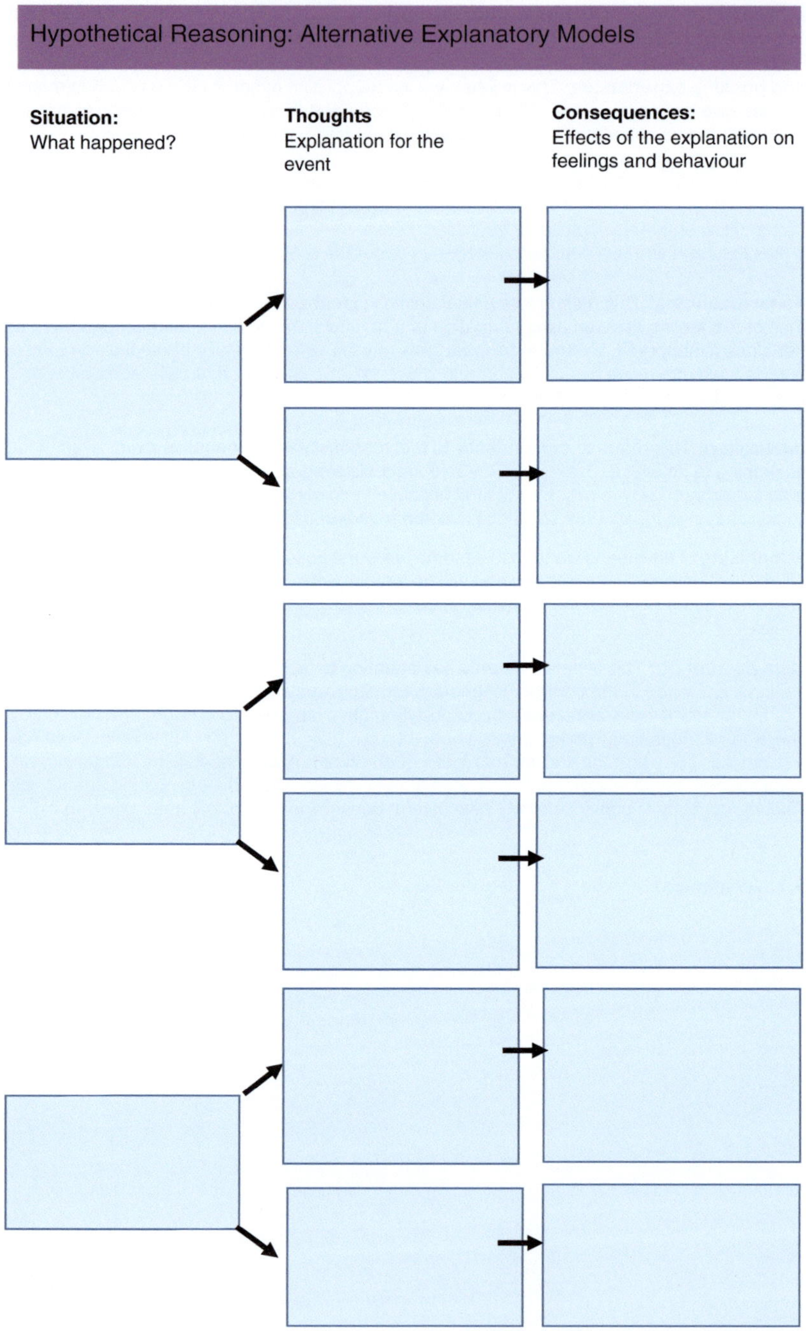

Fig. 6.1 (continued)

Hypothetical Reasoning: Find Alternative Explanations

Most events have more than one explanation. However, we tend to make the mistake of focusing on only one possible explanation. Check and challenge your thoughts and interpretations. What other assumptions are there that might also explain a particular situation? How likely is it that your initial explanation is actually correct?

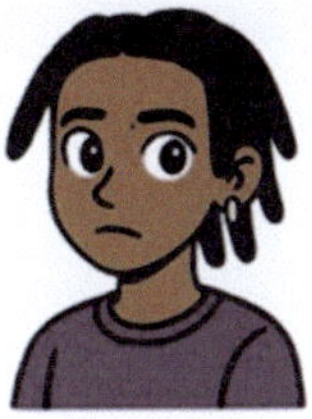

1. What is the situation? (who, what, when, where)?

2. What automatic assumptions did you make in the situation?

3. How did you feel about it?

4. What other explanations have you considered and what feelings have arisen as a result?

-

-

-

5. Which assumptions do you think are the most likely?

Fig. 6.1 (continued)

6. Check the various explanations by looking for evidence and counter-evidence:

Explanation 1
Evidence:

Counter-evidence:

Explanation 2
Evidence:

Counter-evidence:

Explanation 3
Evidence:

Counter-evidence:

Fig. 6.1 (continued)

Everyday Activation

7

An important part of treatment for adolescents meeting CHR criteria is to improve their everyday activation. Many patients describe severe social withdrawal. They lack motivation and feel exhausted quickly, causing them to react by avoiding all demands and activities. Building up positive activities is therefore essential. If patients can be engaged in more activities that are good for them, they usually report an improvement in their state of mind.

At the end of the chapter, the worksheets contain a list of suggestions for positive activities. The positive activities are divided into the categories of physical exercise, creative activities, cognitive training, social interactions, wellness, rewards, and relaxation. Suggestions are thereby pre-formulated, and there is no need to brainstorm activities during the therapy session. Instead, the suggestions can be discussed with the patient during the therapy session, and the patient can merely select which activities to try for the next session. The list also includes activities that most young people do every day anyway, such as taking a shower. The aim of the list, however, is to get patients to treat themselves to a shower (perhaps with a special, nice-smelling shower gel) as a way of caring for themselves. Of course, patients can also add their own ideas to the lists.

Supplementary Information The online version contains supplementary material available at https://doi.org/10.1007/978-3-032-10341-3_7. The videos can be accessed individually by clicking the DOI link in the accompanying figure caption or by scanning this link with the SN More Media App.

N. Traber-Walker, M. Franscini, *Adolescents at Clinical High Risk for Psychosis*,
https://doi.org/10.1007/978-3-032-10341-3_7

Initially, we recommend encouraging patients to do at least one positive activity a day. Later, the goal can be increased to several positive activities per day. Patients should assess their mood before and after doing the activity. This will help them to become more aware of their ability to influence their mood through behavior (see Worksheet "Mood Protocol").

The worksheets also include a weekly planner that can be used in therapy to help young patients organize their daily lives. The weekly schedule can be particularly helpful for young people without a daily structure. Alternatively, it can be used to help structure a busy day. Study time, wellness time, or so-called me time can be included in the weekly planner. In addition to the worksheets for everyday activation, the worksheet "Weekly Goals" (see explanations in Sect. 3.4.2) can be combined with the weekly schedule.

The worksheet "How Can I Stay Healthy?" summarizes the most important elements of a balanced daily routine. Patients can check off what they have done each day.

Positive Everyday Activities

The list of positive activities is also included in the smartphone app Robin Z. There, the categories are the same as those described on the worksheets. Patients can also create their own activities and store them in Robin Z. In the logbook, patients have the opportunity to mark completed positive activities.

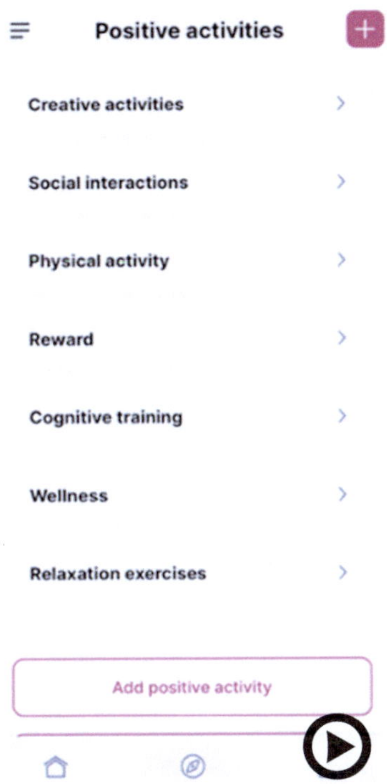

Fig. 7.1 Tutorial video “Library” (▶ https://doi.org/10.1007/000-k5m)

Further explanations on the use of “positive activities” in the therapy session can be found in the tutorial video “**Library**” (Fig. 7.1).

The “Weekly Goals” function offers further support in everyday activation; more information on this can be found in the tutorial video “**Weekly Goals**” (Fig. 7.2).

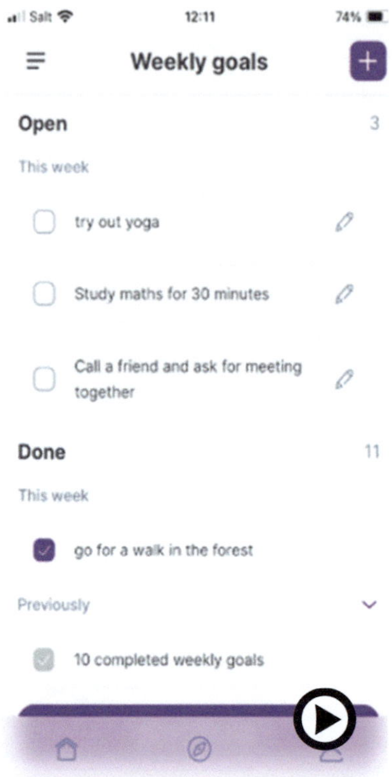

Fig. 7.2 Tutorial video "Weekly Goals" (▶ https://doi.org/10.1007/000-k5k)

7.1 Cognitive Training

The category of 'cognitive training' was intentionally included in the positive activities to emphasize that practicing cognitive skills need not necessarily be seen as something demanding, stressful, or boring. Regular practice helps to improve cognitive performance and can be employed in cognitive remediation computer programs, ideal for training cognitive skills. In order for the learning effect to be sustainable, it is advisable to regularly test the skills in different contexts of everyday life. However, the patient's motivation to engage with these topics is a fundamental prerequisite.

This leads to the following questions:

What do I want to achieve? What is my short-term goal, and what is my long-term goal?

Motivation for regular cognitive training can be very low if the only reason for practicing is to improve academic performance. In order to find the individual motivation for this time-consuming practice, a careful analysis of short and long-term goals is recommended.

What should I learn or practice in order to achieve this goal?

Making a good choice of exercises and learning material increases the likelihood of success.

Which strategies/techniques can help me to implement my cognitive training in my daily life?

Adaptation of the home environment and use of assistive tools in daily life can contribute to success.

Therapeutic Conversation with Michael

Michael is often unable to concentrate at all. Focusing and concentrating on work has never been easy for him, and now he can barely read a full page. However, with the help of medication, he has been able to achieve the required academic performance. Even so, his memory has become weaker. When he manages to concentrate and read a text, he often doesn't remember exactly what he read a short time later. He noticed the first changes about a year ago. Sometimes Michael's flow of thought is slow, hard, and laborious. Then his mind seems to race so fast that he can't keep up. His thoughts jump from one point to the next. This racing mind often ends in total chaos. There is so much going on in his head that he can't follow his own thoughts.

Therapist:	In the last session, we talked at length about the various difficulties you have with your ability to think. We also talked about your increasing avoidance of studying for school.
Michael:	Yes, but not because I'm lazy. I just get so frustrated. I can't study properly. I can't concentrate well enough to read. If I do manage a few minutes of concentration, I can't remember whatever I've read or concentrated on after I finish.
Therapist:	We have already discussed the possibility of using computer programs to train certain thinking skills. However, such training is very time-consuming and requires regular time and practice. Would you be motivated to do this?
Michael:	I'm not sure. But what I know for sure is that I can't go on like this. If things stay the same, I won't make it through vocational school.
Therapist:	So, vocational school is important to you?
Michael:	Well, I don't want to have to repeat the year. In order to do that, I need to get good grades at school. So I need to get these thinking problems under control.
Therapist:	Are there any other areas of your life, apart from vocational school, where better thinking skills would be important?
Michael:	Well, I want to get my driving license, and that requires concentration. Plus, I tend to get distracted during conversations, or my thoughts slow down so much that I can't follow the conversation. I don't think anyone has noticed that yet.
Therapist:	If I understand you correctly, you would like to improve your thinking so that you can continue your apprenticeship, learn to drive a car, and feel more confident in conversations with other people.
Michael:	(nods) yes. There might be more reasons, but I can't think of them now.

Therapist:	These are very good and important reasons. Shall we write them down on your exercise sheet under number one?
Michael:	(nods)
Therapist:	My next question is: In order to achieve your goals, what skill might you work on in training?
Michael:	Hmmm. My memory, I think, and being less distracted.
Therapist:	I think it would be a good start to do exercises to improve your memory and work on focusing your attention. Can you think of anything that could help you in your daily life? Any tools or skills? Perhaps we could start by focusing your attention and being less distracted. Do you remember what worked in school previously to help you not get distracted?
Michael:	I had already worked out a few things with my teacher. I used to sit in the front row, so I could only see the teacher. And when I was reading a text, I always held my ruler under the current line so that I didn't slip into the text and leave something out.
Therapist:	I think those are two very important hints. When you're studying, choose a place where you won't be disturbed and have few distractions, such as facing a wall. I like the idea of the ruler. Couldn't that help you when you have to read a text for school?

The following sections contain some suggestions on how cognitive training can be applied in everyday life.

7.1.1 Pack a Bag for a School Day

At first glance, this task sounds simple and relatively unimportant. However, it involves several cognitive challenges and requires some planning. The aim is to carry all the essentials for the school day without packing the bag too heavily.

Questions to consider include:

- What subjects do I have tomorrow, and what do I need for them?
- What will I be doing after school? What do I need for that?
- What's the weather forecast for tomorrow? Do I need an umbrella, sunglasses, or an extra jumper?

Packing a bag should become a daily routine that is done without procrastination. It can be helpful to combine it with another daily routine.

7.1.2 Grocery Shopping

Grocery shopping can be an easy way to train memory skills. Young patients should be encouraged to look at their shopping list only at the end and try to find all the ingredients without a list. When weighing fruit or vegetables, several numbers can be remembered at the same time, e.g., oranges equal number 33, apples equal number 71, and onions equal number 59. The number of numbers that patients have to remember at one time can be increased gradually.

Adding up prices in one's head before paying helps to avoid nasty bills and is a good way to practice math skills.

7.1.3 Reading Training

Regular reading is one of the most effective ways to train various cognitive skills. The complexity of what is read is less important. Patients should choose a text that interests them. This could be a novel, a short story, or an article from a magazine. Articles from teen magazines are also suitable.

For patients with concentration problems, reading training should start with the shortest possible units. Five minutes a day may be enough to start. Reading time should be increased each week. If possible, the first exercise session should take place during the therapy session. This involves the patient telling the therapist in a few key words what they have just read. This step is important in order to refute negative thoughts such as "I can't remember anything anyway. My thinking doesn't work anymore." During reading training at home, the patient should write down a few key words each day and give a rough summary of the reading material at the next therapy session.

Therapeutic Conversation with Lucy

Lucy:	At school, I have to read this book. I used to love reading. I used to read books straight away, sometimes a whole book in a day. Now I can barely read a chapter. It's so frustrating.
Therapist:	That sounds very exhausting. Do you have any idea why that is?
Lucy:	Well, I just can't concentrate properly anymore. Sometimes I'll read a page, but I can't really take in what I'm reading. It's like my brain is full of holes, and the words are slipping through.
Therapist:	That's very well phrased. A lot of young people who come here talk about problems like that. I think it's particularly difficult for you because you used to find it easy to read, learn, and concentrate.
Lucy:	Yes, I don't understand it. I also have the feeling that it's getting worse.
Therapist:	Is there anything you are trying to do about it?
Lucy:	Well, I don't read any more unless I absolutely have to. Only things for school, but it's not easy.
Therapist:	The problem with this strategy, which is called avoidance, is that it doesn't really help in the long run. You are avoiding a book you want to read. You may be less frustrated at the moment, but your reading skills will decline. This happens very quickly. And reading becomes more and more associated with an unpleasant experience for you. Your subconscious records this as "reading = very unpleasant, avoid if possible," and over time, even as "reading = impossible." so the mere thought of having to read something makes you feel uncomfortable. Do you understand what I'm saying?
Lucy:	I think I do. Before I even start, I feel like I won't be able to concentrate anyway.
Therapist:	The good news is that you can practice your reading skills again. If you think back to first grade, you couldn't read fluently, and it was hard at first. After a while, it wasn't so hard.
Lucy:	You mean I have to learn to read all over again?

Therapist:	(smiles) no, of course not. You need to practice reading longer texts. Experience that you actually enjoy reading. Your reading ability is there. You can still read. It's more a question of concentration and focus.
Lucy:	And how can I practice this?
Therapist:	I'd say choose a book that you find particularly exciting or interesting, one that you think you'll enjoy reading. Then read it for ten minutes straight, every day. After ten minutes, you can put it down, but first concentrate for those ten minutes.
Lucy:	I don't get very far in ten minutes anymore.
Therapist:	That's okay. You're looking for a place to start so that you can grow, and this is the place. Over time, it will get easier. Then, you'll be able to extend your reading time to 15 minutes or 20 minutes, etc.

7.1.4 Playing Games

Playing games is fun and also trains attention, concentration, memory, and flexible thinking. Patients can play alone, in pairs, or in groups. There are also various computer games that train cognitive skills.

Below are some game recommendations, organized by skill, that train important cognitive abilities.

- Attention, concentration, perception: I Spy, Jenga, Mastermind.
- Organizing, categorizing: Dominoes, Rummy, Uno.
- Processing speed: Speed, Spot It, Jungle Speed.
- (Working) Memory: Memory, Sudoku.
- Change of perspective: Dixit, Werewolf, Codenames.

Playing in a group encourages communication and community. Though family play is very common among younger children, parents often stop playing with their children when they reach their teens. However, family game nights have a very positive impact on family life. During family sessions in therapy, it can be suggested to organize game nights together, and it should be mentioned that these games have a positive effect on the patient's everyday functioning. A game night can be divided into three courses, similar to a fancy dinner: At the beginning is the starter, a short warm-up game (with simple rules lasting no more than 10 minutes). Then the actual evening game takes the role of the main course (with a duration of approximately 45 minutes) and, for the final game, dessert (cooling down with simple rules and lasting no longer than 10 minutes).

A few examples:

- Warm-up games: Speed, Spot it, Blink, Tenzi.
- Evening games: Dixit, Carcassonne, Codenames.
- Final games: Simon Says, Take 5, Uno.

Alternatively, each family member can choose a game to play.

7.2 Creative Activities

Engaging in creative activities offers a range of benefits that enrich daily life and contribute to personal development. Creative activities stimulate new and different ways of thinking. Immersing oneself in creative tasks encourages thinking outside the box, leading to innovative solutions and fresh perspectives.

During creative acts, patients train their cognitive skills by using important thinking processes such as working memory, focusing attention, or executive functions. This happens unconsciously and spontaneously, which is why creative activities are generally perceived as less stressful than, for example, completing schoolwork. Since it carries less stress and still exercises cognitive functions, creativity is especially useful for cognitive remediation. Physical benefits are also notable; activities such as painting, sculpting, or playing an instrument can improve fine motor skills and hand-eye coordination.

Completing creative projects provides a sense of accomplishment, which boosts self-confidence and self-esteem. They are a powerful means of self-expression, allowing individuals to communicate their thoughts, feelings, and identities in unique and meaningful ways. Therefore, creative activities can provide alternatives for moments of success, especially for adolescents experiencing cognitive decline in academic performance.

Creativity is a broad term, and practically everyone enjoys some kind of creative activity. It includes drawing, playing an instrument, cooking, baking, gardening, and other activities. Patients should be encouraged to try several activities to find out what suits them.

Below are some examples of how different creative activities can be applied in therapy.

7.2.1 Planting Flowers

Planting and caring for flowers involves several components that are important for daily functioning. Planting itself provides new tactile experiences: How does the soil feel? How do the seeds feel? It is also a motor activity that requires sensitivity. During a therapy session with the patient, flower seeds can be planted in a small pot. The pot is then taken home.

Taking care of a plant requires a certain amount of responsibility. It is not enough just to sow the seeds; the seeds have to be watered, and the patient must look after the plant, seeing that it gets the necessary light and nutrients. The patient has to take care of the plant, or it will not grow.

When selecting seeds, look for a plant that will grow in a reasonably short amount of time so that the first green leaves can be seen after a week or two.

7.2.2 Music

Patients who play an instrument can be encouraged to play regularly in front of their parents or friends. Whenever possible, they should try to learn the piece by heart, which will train their memory. The steps involved can be discussed during therapy:

- Which piece of music should I choose?
- How much time do I need to master the piece?
- How will I structure my practice?
- When would be a suitable date to perform in front of the family?

7.2.3 Invitation to Dinner

Both cooking and baking are very effective ways of training cognitive functions. It starts with preparation. A recipe is chosen, and a shopping list is made.

Patients who enjoy trying out recipes should be encouraged to cook for family or friends. This is a great opportunity for positive social interaction and a chance to receive praise and recognition for the effort made. The patient does not need to handle the entire meal alone, but the cooking can be done together or by dividing up the dishes among different people. Planning a dinner event is another exercise in cognitive skills.

How to proceed with the planning can be discussed in advance in the therapy session.

- When and whom do I invite?
- Which recipe(s) do I choose?
- What do I need to have to make this recipe? Where can I get the ingredients and other supplies?
- Plan the cooking process: How do I start? How long will each step take? What should I prepare first, and what next?
- What tasks can I delegate? Who can help with table decorations or tidying up?

7.2.4 Craft Activities

Other patients have a talent for arts and crafts, knitting, or sewing. All of these activities are ideal for implementing cognitive remediation in everyday life. They require planning skills both in preparation and in realization. The preparation phase involves finding suitable instructions, for example, a basic sewing pattern for a dress. The Internet can be used as a research tool for some ideas. Another option is to look at dresses in shops to get an idea of the type of dress to make. The next step is to collect the appropriate materials.

Whatever type of creative activity the adolescent chooses, it is useful to discuss each step in therapy in order to make it work.

Therapeutic Conversation with Michael

Therapist:	You say that lately you never feel like doing anything.
Michael:	Yes, I used to have a lot of hobbies, but not anymore. Since I stopped playing football, I just hang around a lot. My apprenticeship is also very stressful, so of course, I have less spare time.
Therapist:	What were your hobbies before?
Michael:	Football, as I said. And meeting people. I still enjoy playing football, but I have less time. Also, I'm tired after work and don't feel like going out to see anyone.
Therapist:	Are there any other things you like to do? Things that don't take up much time? Or that you could do alone, without having to meet friends first?
Michael:	Well, I used to have a lot of fun drawing comics.
Therapist:	Why did you stop?
Michael:	I have no idea. At some point, my sketchpad was full, and I just stopped. It was around the time I started my apprenticeship.
Therapist:	Would you like to start drawing again?
Michael:	I think so, yes.
Therapist:	When did you last draw?
Michael:	On holiday with my parents. I watched some people on the street outside the restaurant and did some sketches of them on a napkin. They were quite good. But I left them in the hotel.
Therapist:	Could you see yourself drawing more comics again?
Michael:	I would have to get a sketchpad again first.
Therapist:	So that would be the first step? Buying a sketchpad?
Michael:	Two, a big one for at home and a small one so I can sketch ideas on the go.
Therapist:	That sounds like a very good idea.
Michael:	For me, too, actually. Maybe I could even sketch on my way to work.
Therapist:	What else do you need to get back to drawing?
Michael:	The right pens, of course. But I'm sure they're still in my room. I just have to find them.
Therapist:	Would it be a good idea to get two sketch pads and find the pens by next week?

7.3 Physical Activity

It is generally known that exercise has a positive effect on physical and mental well-being. Even people without mental health problems generally feel fitter, more alert, and more productive when they exercise than when they do not. Several studies have shown a link between physical activity and a reduction in psychotic and depressive symptoms.

Most kids enjoy movement and physical activity, but regular physical activity tends to decrease during adolescence. Sports activities are often given up. These hobbies are time-consuming and often incompatible with the demands of school or work. Another reason may be that interests change, and a particular activity is suddenly no longer enjoyable.

The benefits of exercise are obvious. Practically all sports require cognitive skills as well as physical performance. Sports such as dancing, aerobics, yoga, or martial arts train memory, as certain sequences of movements have to be memorized. Ball sports, on the other hand, train the ability to focus attention. Some patients meeting CHR criteria also have impaired motor skills. Many sports help to improve gross motor skills and, in particular, coordination.

Team sports are also good for developing social skills. In general, sports provide opportunities for social interaction and meeting new people. By joining a new club, it is easier to make new social contacts than in other places because there are already common interests.

For adolescents treated with antipsychotics, physical activity also helps to counteract pharmacologically induced weight gain.

The category of physical activity within positive activities aims to motivate patients to take more exercise in their daily lives. There are suggestions not only for physically active patients but also for those who are reluctant to exercise.

Each activity must be adapted to the current level of fitness. In particular, patients who often feel tired and drained should still be encouraged to do more exercise. It does not have to be a marathon. Even taking the stairs or getting off the bus one stop earlier and walking the rest of the way home can make a difference. A 15-minute walk outside increases physical and mental well-being. Some patients will feel an added sense of achievement in the activity or in keeping a diary of daily physical activity. Smartphone apps such as pedometers are also helpful.

Therapeutic Conversation with Lucy

Lucy:	I'm so exhausted and tired. Luckily I don't have any exams this week. So for once I don't have to study today.
Therapist:	That's great; I can imagine it's a relief. What are you going to do instead?
Lucy:	Honestly? I'd like to go straight home, get into bed, and just fall asleep.
Therapist:	Hm, do you think that's a good idea?
Lucy:	I know it's not a good idea. We've talked about this many times.
Therapist:	Is there anything else you want to do?
Lucy:	Not really. I just want to lie down and do nothing.
Therapist:	Let's have a quick look at your list of positive activities. Maybe you can think of something? Which category do you think would be most appropriate?
Lucy:	Wellness!
Therapist:	(smiles) good. Then have a look at the wellness suggestions. Is there anything you would like to do?
Lucy:	I might like to go to the sauna. There's a sauna and a steam room at my gym.
Therapist:	That's a great idea. Do you go to the sauna often?
Lucy:	Not as often as I used to. I don't exercise much anymore, and it feels strange to go to the gym just to have a sauna. Nobody else does that. Actually, the sauna is always the reward for having worked out before.
Therapist:	Can you still imagine going there and just using the sauna?
Lucy:	Not really.
Therapist:	How about a workout and then a sauna?
Lucy:	I'm too exhausted. I just can't do an hour's training today.
Therapist:	An hour is a long time. What's your favorite piece of equipment at the gym?
Lucy:	The cross trainer, which works both legs and arms. I usually spend half an hour on the elliptical and then do some weightlifting.
Therapist:	An hour of exercise is quite a long time. How long would you last on the cross trainer at the moment?
Lucy:	No time at all.
Therapist:	I don't think so. Not even five minutes?
Lucy:	Well, five minutes. Anyone can do that.
Therapist:	How about ten minutes?

Lucy:	Yes, I can do ten minutes.
Therapist:	Ten minutes is quite a lot, I think. Ten minutes on the elliptical makes a big difference. It's a third of the time you normally spend on the cross trainer.
Lucy:	Hm, I don't know.
Therapist:	How much have you been training the last few days?
Lucy:	I haven't been.
Therapist:	So ten minutes on the elliptical would be ten minutes more than you exercised all week.
Lucy:	Yes, that's right.
Therapist:	And then you go to the sauna. How does that sound? Do you think that would be possible?
Lucy:	Yes, I should be able to do that. Ten minutes isn't that long. I could do that. Maybe even more.
Therapist:	Of course you can do more. But if you've had enough after ten minutes, you can always stop.
Lucy:	And then go to the sauna! I'll try it.
Therapist:	How do you think you'll feel after ten minutes on the cross trainer and then a sauna?
Lucy:	Probably even more tired. But a different kind of tired. A good tiredness.

7.4 Social Interactions

Many adolescents with CHR symptoms report problems with social interactions. Social contacts should always be well explored during the diagnostic phase, and social withdrawal should be addressed by the therapist. If patients report that they tend to be loners and have always enjoyed spending time alone, the therapist needs to be aware that this may not be entirely true. Peer relationships are particularly important during adolescence. It is possible that patients have come to terms with their social isolation. However, clinical experience shows that this loneliness is usually only partly voluntary. If patients manage to develop their social skills and make friends during the course of therapy, they almost always report feeling better and that the previous state of being alone was not really satisfying.

It is important to ask about the underlying reasons for withdrawal:

- Are they withdrawing because they no longer feel socially skilled?
- Are they embarrassed and ashamed of their CHR symptoms?
- Are they being excluded or rejected by peers?
- Is withdrawal associated with negative symptoms or depression, such as lethargy and exhaustion?
- Is there some social anxiety that leads to avoidance of interactions?
- Is the withdrawal caused by paranoid thoughts or distrust of others?

The recommended therapeutic approach depends on the reason for social withdrawal. When patients have a good social network and feel integrated but have withdrawn because of their symptoms, therapy should discuss how they can maintain their friendships despite their withdrawal. Me-time (such as contact-free or mobile-free time) is a vital component in stressful moments and experiences of overwhelm, but it is important that patients who tend toward social isolation still be encouraged to make social appointments. For example, instead of cancelling, they should attend social engagements despite feeling tired and simply stay for less time.

In times of crisis, social contact may be limited to close friends and those who can cope with the fact that the patient is not doing so well. However, other acquaintances should not be neglected too much. Social media is a particularly good way to stay in touch. There, patients should respond to requests. They can say that they are too busy at the moment to keep in touch regularly, but it is important that they respond to contact requests, no matter how exhausted they are. In therapy, responses to requests from distant friends can be discussed together. Distancing can be practiced. Excuses such as "I have a lot of exams at the moment" are perfectly acceptable. Once patients are feeling better, it is important that their social contacts are still available and that they are able to socialize again.

Patients who have few or no social contacts should be supported to (re)build a social network. Who are they most likely to socialize with? Do they have classmates they get on with? Is there someone from their past they could reconnect with? Maybe someone in the neighborhood?

Social media sites such as Facebook, Snapchat, and Instagram offer many opportunities to make new contacts or reconnect with old friends. The Internet can also be a way for socially insecure young people to make new friends and connect with others. This can be used as an opportunity. Writing a message on social media is much easier than making a phone call.

It is useful to discuss each step in detail during therapy. Which of their friends and followers on social media could be contacted? The first step might be liking pictures without leaving a comment. This is something that even socially insecure adolescents dare to do. As a second step, perhaps after the other person has also liked one of their pictures, a comment could be left. This will increase the chances of getting in touch. Alternatively, if patients feel confident enough, they can send a private message directly to the person in question.

The topic of arranging meetings with friends should be given a lot of space in therapy. The first step is to decide who is to be approached. What kind of appointment is proposed? Do they have a common interest in a certain film, music group, or sport?

Another option, particularly suitable for classmates, is to ask about studying together. During therapy, role-playing can be used to practice approaching peers and making appointments.

Therapeutic Conversation with Michael

Michael has not yet managed to make friends at his vocational school.

Michael:	At the beginning of the school year, I often didn't feel so well, so I didn't really fit in. Now a lot of friendships have already formed, and I don't really fit in.
Therapist:	It's understandable that this situation is not easy for you. Is there anyone in your class that you get on with? Who do you spend your breaks with?
Michael:	I'm often with a large group, but I don't really take part in the conversations. Last Monday I had lunch alone again because I had to ask the teacher a question. The group had already left. I knew where they were going, but I didn't dare to join them.
Therapist:	And you could have gone afterward, right?
Michael:	Probably. I don't really know.
Therapist:	In this large group, is there anyone you like? Perhaps someone with whom you've had a longer conversation?
Michael:	There are two people I really get on with: Dave and Luca. The three of us did a group project once, and that went well.
Therapist:	But you've never connected outside of school?
Michael:	Once, because of the group work. But not otherwise.
Therapist:	Do you think you could meet them both, or even one at a time?
Michael:	I can. But I'm really afraid to ask. I feel so stupid. What am I supposed to say? Would either of you like to be my school friend?
Therapist:	It's not an easy situation, I know. But what can you lose?
Michael:	I'm afraid I'll make a fool of myself, that they'll say no, and I'll feel rejected.
Therapist:	Do you have anything in common? Like the same football team you like? Or a band whose concert you would like to go to?
Michael:	Hm, I can't think of anything right now. I don't know them well enough to meet them outside of school.
Therapist:	You made friends on the sports team, didn't you? That was about the same time.
Michael:	Yes, but it was easier somehow. There are only three of us who are about my age. We had lunch together several times, so that's why we were friends.
Therapist:	Would it be possible for you to have lunch with Dave and Luca? Instead of in the whole group?
Michael:	(thinking) maybe I could. Yes. Luca has actually already pointed out several times that he doesn't like the takeaway where we always go.
Therapist:	Might you make a suggestion for lunch? Is there a restaurant you know that would be suitable?
Michael:	I ate alone last time. I walked in the other direction to make sure I didn't bump into anyone from class, and then I found a bakery that had good sandwiches. I could suggest that.
Therapist:	That would be an idea. Do you know how you could bring that into conversation?
Michael:	(thinking for a moment) I could mention that I've been to this bakery with really good sandwiches. So I could ask Luca if he would like to go there instead of the takeaway. He usually sits next to Dave, so I could say it so they both hear.
Therapist:	Do you think you could do that?
Michael:	Maybe. I think it would be possible.

The possibility of rejection should be anticipated in the preparatory discussion. It is important to point out that rejection does not necessarily have anything to do with the person. Every contact is considered a success. The next peer may say yes, and it is usually easier to ask again.

Patients meeting CHR criteria tend to take rejection very personally and may even develop a paranoid reaction to it. It is therefore recommended that this issue be addressed in therapy, along with a detailed conversation about possible rejection and cancellation.

Therapeutic Conversation with Lucy

Lucy comes to her therapy session feeling depressed. Over the past few months, Lucy has become increasingly socially withdrawn, rarely seeing her friends, but recently she has been trying to socialize again. She reports that, last Friday, none of her friends wanted to hang out with her, and she feels rejected as a result.

Lucy:	I feel like ever since I started trying to see my friends again, all I get is rejection. Sometimes I feel like they're all against me and don't really want to be friends with me anymore.
Therapist:	I'm sorry to hear that, Lucy.
Lucy:	Even my two best friends never have time for me.
Therapist:	Hm, that surprises me. They've made such an effort to keep in touch with you.
Lucy:	I think maybe they don't want to be friends anymore, but they can't bring themselves to say so. Instead, they always have an excuse or other plans.
Therapist:	Can you describe a situation in which your friends didn't want to go out with you?
Lucy:	Last Friday, I asked Jamie if she wanted to go to the cinema with me that evening. She said she was meeting her cousin. That sounds like a lame excuse to me.
Therapist:	Why do you think that is an excuse?
Lucy:	Well, it's just a feeling.
Therapist:	You said that your two closest friends no longer want to see you. What about the other one?
Lucy:	After Jamie said she already had plans, I didn't dare ask anyone else. I was too scared of another rejection when even Jamie found an excuse not to meet me.
Therapist:	Lucy, I want to ask you again, why are you so sure it was an excuse?
Lucy:	Well, like I said, it's just a feeling. I haven't felt well all week. Then on Friday I felt a bit better. I felt more energetic and spontaneously wanted to go out. After Jamie rejected me, I felt much worse. Then I suddenly had the feeling that Jamie was against me. I can't explain it; like I said, it's just a feeling.
Therapist:	Let us look at this situation again. When exactly on Friday did you ask Jamie to go to the cinema with you?
Lucy:	After school, around 4 pm.
Therapist:	Does Jamie usually stay at home on Friday evenings?
Lucy:	No, of course not. She usually goes out on Fridays. I used to, too, but not lately because I was always so exhausted.
Therapist:	Is it not possible that Jamie had already made an appointment with her cousin?
Lucy:	Well, maybe. I guess it was Friday already, and it could have been short notice for her. We usually plan our weekends at the beginning of the week.
Therapist:	What do you think? Would it be better to ask a few days earlier next time if you want to do something on the weekend?
Lucy:	Hm, maybe I could try that.

7.5 Wellness and Reward

As described in previous chapters, effective stress management is a key factor in preventing the transition to psychosis. The categories of wellness and rewards should help one to recover from stressful everyday life. In addition, regular use of these activities can prevent situations of excessive demands.

The wellness category includes ideas on how to consciously take small breaks from everyday life. It is worth taking time with patients to consider what small wellness rituals they can include in their daily routines. These could be activities they do in the evening before going to bed in order to relax and unwind from everyday life.

There is a rewards category in addition to the wellness category, although the two categories may overlap to some extent. The aim of the reward category is to reward oneself for something specific. Patients should be aware of what they have achieved that day and think about what they deserve a reward for. Activities such as gaming, watching TV, or surfing the Internet can be found under the reward category. These are activities that most adolescents often do enough anyway, though they may be doing them with a guilty conscience. "I should be studying, but instead I've watched two more episodes of my favorite soap." Such thoughts are not helpful. The idea of a reward, on the other hand, might lead to the thought, "If I study for half an hour, I can watch my favorite show afterward," or "I've had a very hard day today, so I'm tired now. I'll treat myself to an episode of my favorite show."

Therapeutic Conversation with Lucy

Lucy:	I have so many exams at school this week that I can't do any of the positive activities every day.
Therapist:	I think that's a shame. Especially when you're under so much stress, you should do something for yourself. Take little breaks to relax.
Lucy:	I know. But now it's the last two weeks of term, and I just have to get through. I come home and start studying, then we eat, I study, and then I go to bed.
Therapist:	Do you sleep well when you go to bed right after studying?
Lucy:	Hm, yes. But sometimes it's difficult. I'm exhausted and tired, but somehow I'm not satisfied. Because all day long I've been doing nothing but school and studying.
Therapist:	Exactly, I can understand that. That's what I meant when I said you should take some time for yourself.
	It's not that you need to take a big break. I'm talking about little, everyday breaks, moments in between when you treat yourself to something nice. There are lots of short activities on the list of positive activities that you might have to do anyway. But the point is to do them consciously. Shall we take a closer look at the reward and wellness categories?
Lucy:	(nods and looks at the two worksheets) having a shower or a bath is always an option. So is listening to music.
Therapist:	I think it would be good if you took a short break after school and studied afterward.
Lucy:	Well...
Therapist:	To be honest, Lucy, how long does it usually take you to start studying?
Lucy:	Hm, probably about 15 minutes. Until I've set the table. I wash my hands, have a drink...

Therapist:	Exactly. So you are taking breaks anyway. But I personally think it would be more effective if you consciously set aside a small window of time before you study. 15 minutes to do something you enjoy.
Lucy:	Yeah, maybe.
Therapist:	How about reserving the first 15 minutes for a study-free period? You shouldn't study during those 15 minutes.
Lucy:	Actually, I think that's a good idea.
Therapist:	Instead, you could choose one of the positive activities to do. Agreed?
Lucy:	Agreed.
Therapist:	You should also do something you enjoy in the last 15 minutes before you go to bed. It has been shown that the quality of sleep is better when we have some kind of bedtime ritual. It could be something as simple as taking a warm shower or bath. Or having a cup of tea.
Lucy:	When I was at primary school, my sister and I used to drink a cup of milk before going to bed. It was actually really nice.
Therapist:	Maybe the two of you could start doing it again. I think it would be good for her too.
Lucy:	Yes, I think so too.
Therapist:	We've talked about taking short breaks so you don't have to study all the time. But I think that with the intense program you have now, you can also treat yourself to a reward every now and then. Why don't you think about what you could do for yourself between now and your next session? You can read through the suggestions in the rewards section. Or maybe you have some ideas of your own.

7.6 Worksheets (Fig. 7.3)

- Worksheet 38 "Protocol of Positive Activities".
- Worksheet 39 "Reward".
- Worksheet 40 "Physical Activity".
- Worksheet 41 "Creative Activities".
- Worksheet 42 "Wellness".
- Worksheet 43 "Social Interactions".
- Worksheet 44 "Cognitive Training".
- Worksheet 45 "Relaxation Exercises".
- Worksheet 46 "How Do I Stay Healthy?"
- Worksheet 47 "Weekly Schedule".

Weekly Goals

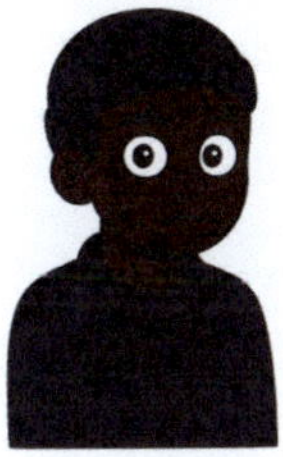

Set three goals for this week. Think of things you would like to do this week. For example, start reading a certain book, or tidy up your room.

1. Goal

Made it:☐

2. Goal

Made it:☐

3. Goal

Made it:☐

Fig. 7.3 Worksheet 38 to Worksheet 47

Protocol of Positive Activities

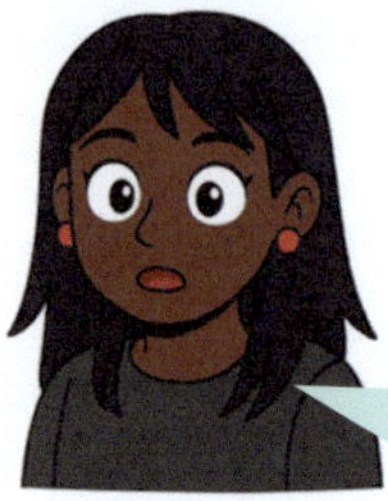

How we feel is closely linked to what we do. Activities that we enjoy automatically make us feel better. It is important to set aside time at least once a day to do something just for yourself. Try to choose at least one suggestion from the list of positive activities every day.

Rate your mood before and after doing the activity from 0 -10:

0= I feel extremely bad

10= I am doing extremely well

——— 2 ——— 4 ——— 6 ——— 8 ——— 10

	Monday	Tuesday	Wednesday	Thursday
Activity				
Mood Before / after	/	/	/	/

	Friday	Saturday	Sunday
Activity			
Mood Before/ after	/	/	/

Fig. 7.3 (continued)

Reward

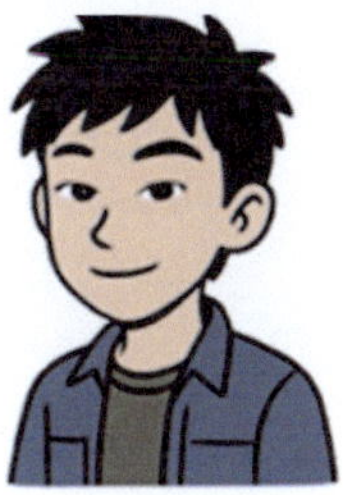

We all deserve rewards, not just for big, extraordinary things. There are reasons to reward ourselves every day, such as getting up and going to school even though we weren't feeling well. Rewarding yourself for what you've done can make a world of difference.

Suggestions:

✓ Download a movie or series
✓ Watch TV
✓ Listen to new music
✓ Eat chocolate
✓ Go out for a meal
✓ Surf the web
✓ Gaming
✓ Try on some nice clothes
✓ Go shopping
✓ Donate to a good cause
✓ Sleep in
✓ Give yourself a present
✓ Visit a place that is full of good memories
✓ Get flowers for yourself
✓ Cook for yourself

Own Ideas:

✓ …

✓ …

✓ …

Fig. 7.3 (continued)

Physical Activities

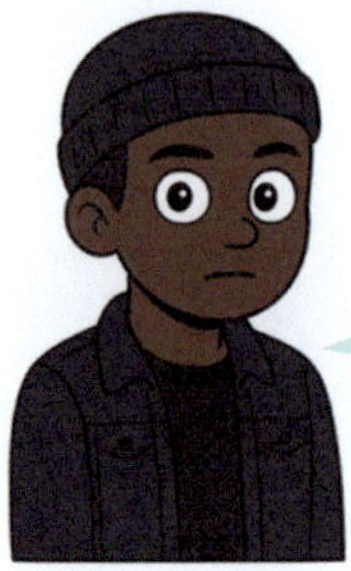

We all know that exercise is important for our health, but we don't always feel motivated to do it. However, it is essential for your health that you get enough movement in your daily life. The type of exercise you do is less important than the fact that you do it. It doesn't have to be intense cardio. What's more important is that you find ways to incorporate physical activity into your daily routine and enjoy it.

Suggestions:

✓ Go for a walk
✓ Go for a run
✓ Dance
✓ Go for a swim
✓ Go rollerblading or ice skating
✓ Ride your bike
✓ Go to a park
✓ Do some sit-ups or push-ups
✓ Play jump rope
✓ Go to a climbing wall
✓ Play hula hoop
✓ Play football
✓ Use stairs instead of the elevator
✓ Get off a bus station earlier and walk the rest of the way
✓ Earn pocket money by walking your neighbour's dog

Own Ideas:

✓ …

✓ …

✓ …

Fig. 7.3 (continued)

Creative Activities

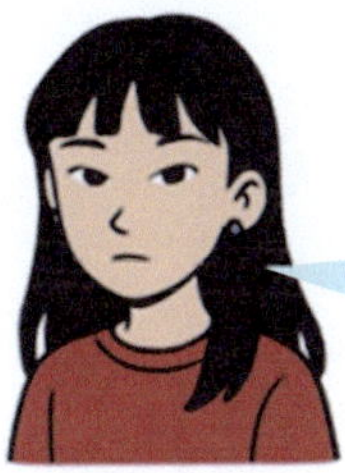

Creative activities provide a vital counterbalance to our intellectually demanding daily lives. They engage different areas of the brain compared to tasks at school or work. Participating in creative activities can help reduce stress and promote a healthy sense of balance in life.

Suggestions:

✓ Singing
✓ Cooking or baking
✓ Writing
✓ Drawing or painting
✓ Colouring a mandala
✓ Playing a musical instrument
✓ Keeping a diary
✓ Writing lyrics to a song
✓ Taking photographs
✓ Planting flowers
✓ Doing make-up or hair
✓ Craftwork
✓ Sewing
✓ Knitting
✓ Creating a collage
✓ Writing a letter to someone
✓ Creating a gift
✓ Rearranging your room
✓ Search for ideas on Pinterest

Own Ideas:

✓ …

✓ …

✓ …

Fig. 7.3 (continued)

Wellness

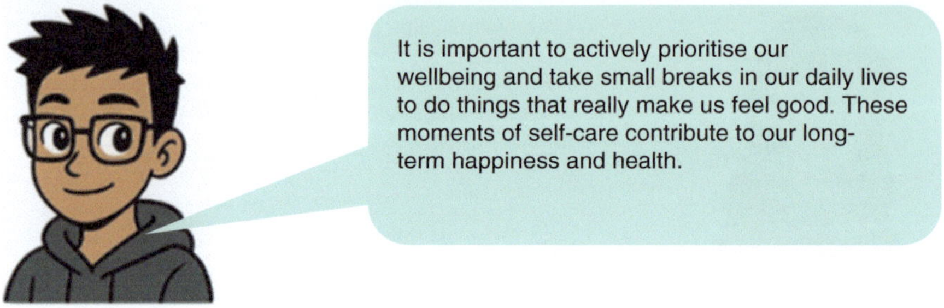

Suggestions:

- ✓ Take a warm bath
- ✓ Get a massage
- ✓ Take a shower
- ✓ Listen to music
- ✓ Lie in the sun
- ✓ Have a tea or coffee
- ✓ Look at photos
- ✓ Go to the sauna or steam room
- ✓ Drink a glass of freshly squeezed orange juice
- ✓ Light a candle

Own Ideas:

- ✓ …
- ✓ …
- ✓ …

Fig. 7.3 (continued)

Social Interactions

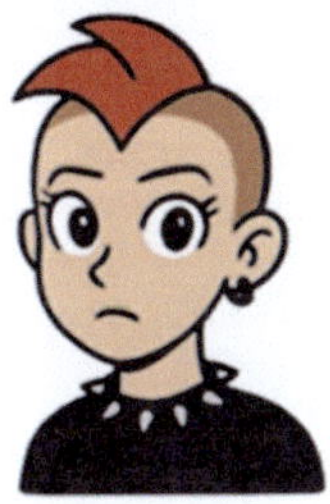

We all have moments when we would rather be alone. Especially when we are not feeling well, we tend to withdraw from others. But socialising is very important for our mental health. Even if you don't feel like it and it takes effort, socialising with your friends, colleagues or family will help you feel better in the long run.

Suggestions

- ✓ Go out with friends
- ✓ Go to the movies
- ✓ Take care of the pets
- ✓ Go to a party
- ✓ Talk to a friend
- ✓ Go for a swim
- ✓ Help someone out
- ✓ Go to a concert
- ✓ Text someone
- ✓ Get in touch with someone you haven't seen to for a long time
- ✓ Play cards
- ✓ Make a phone call
- ✓ Cook for someone
- ✓ Go into the city
- ✓ Go to a mall
- ✓ Have a coffee or tea in a café
- ✓ Invite someone to your home
- ✓ See an exhibition in a museum

Own Ideas:

- ✓ …
- ✓ …
- ✓ …

Fig. 7.3 (continued)

Cognitive Training

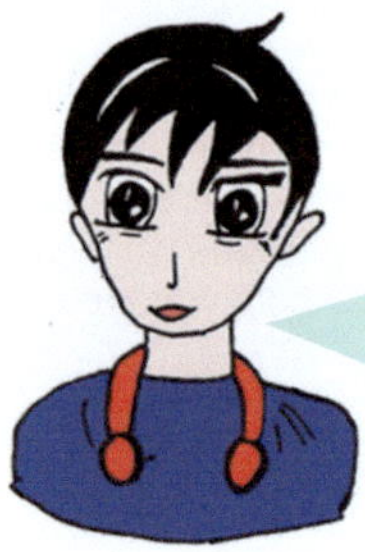

Exercising our brain is essential to keep it in good form, otherwise it will eventually get rusty. This is especially important when we're not feeling our best and notice that our thinking isn't as focused or that we're performing worse at school or other activities. We can improve our cognitive skills by doing exercises. Cognitive training doesn't have to be too exhausting or time-consuming.

Suggestions:

- ✓ Read for 10 minutes
- ✓ Do a puzzle
- ✓ Play a memory game
- ✓ Learn five new words in a foreign language
- ✓ Sudoku
- ✓ Solve a crossword puzzle
- ✓ Count backwards from 20 to 0 in a foreign language
- ✓ Recite the multiplication tables
- ✓ Sing a song and try to learn the verses
- ✓ Watch a movie in a foreign language
- ✓ Learn a dance

Own Ideas:

- ✓ ...
- ✓ ...
- ✓ ...

Fig. 7.3 (continued)

Relaxation Exercises

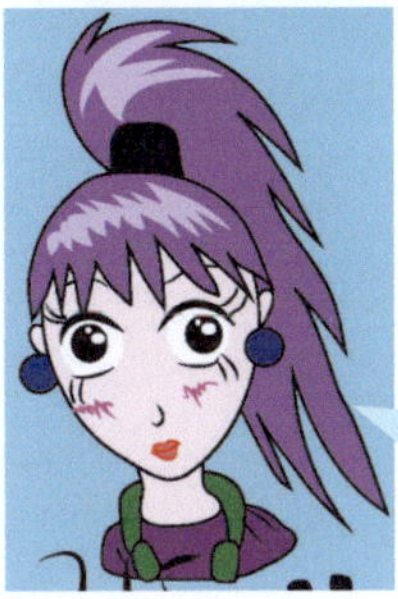

Relaxation helps to release muscle tension and is closely linked to our mental wellbeing. There are several relaxation techniques that can improve how we feel in our bodies. By regularly incorporating relaxation exercises into our daily routine, we can improve our long-term wellbeing and cope better with stress. Here are some suggested relaxation techniques. Instructions for these techniques can be found online, for example on YouTube.

Suggestions:

- ✓ Mindfulness
- ✓ Progressive Muscle Relaxation (PMR)
- ✓ Tai Chi
- ✓ Yoga
- ✓ Autogenic training
- ✓ Qi Gong
- ✓ Feldenkrais

Own Ideas:

- ✓ …
- ✓ …
- ✓ …

Fig. 7.3 (continued)

How Do I Stay Healthy?

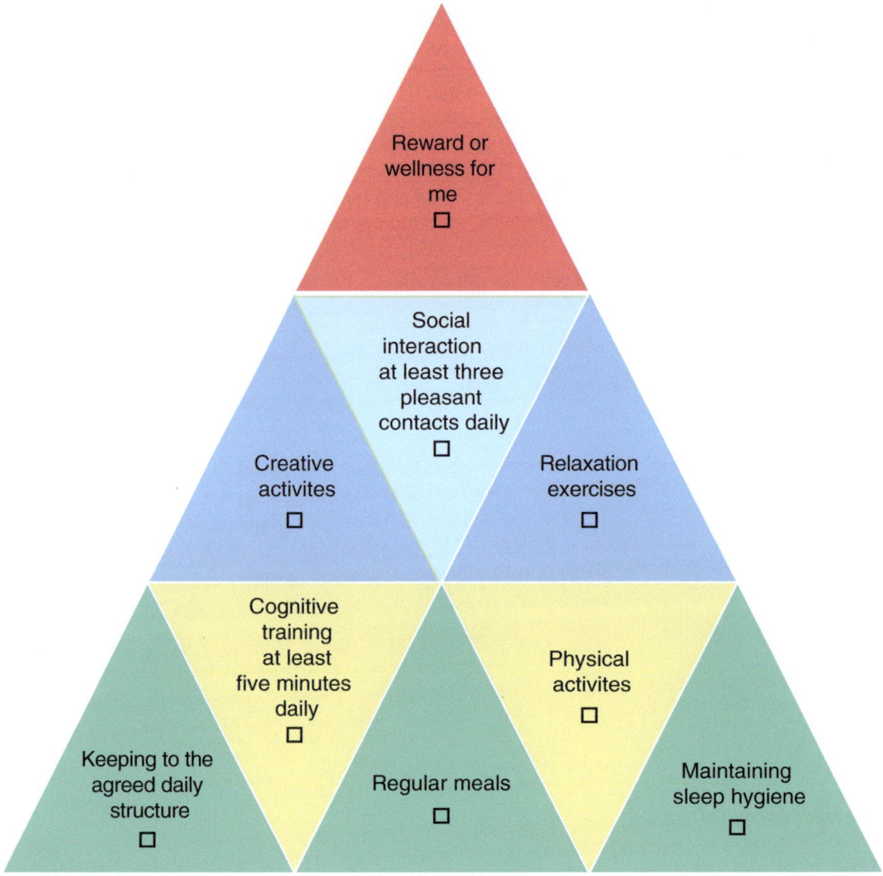

Fig. 7.3 (continued)

Weekly Schedule

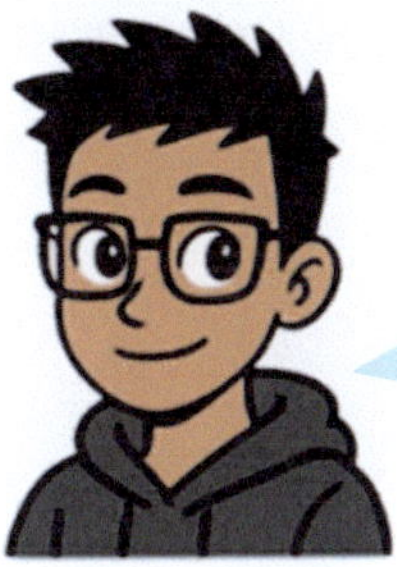

Create a to-do list of activities you want to do this week and try to find time for them alongside your regular daily routine. Be sure to include positive activities in your schedule, such as wellness practices, exercise, or seeing friends.

	Monday	Tuesday	Wednesday	Thursday	Friday	Saturday	Sunday
8:00							
9:00							
10:00							
11:00							
12:00							
13:00							
14:00							
15:00							
16:00							
17:00							
18:00							
19:00							
20:00							
21:00							
22:00							

Fig. 7.3 (continued)

Further Reading

Medalia S. Does cognitive remediation for schizophrenia improve functional outcomes? Curr Opin Psychiatry. 2013;26:151–7.

Medalia B. Cognitive remediation to improve functional outcomes. Oxford: Oxford University Press; 2015.

Roder M. INT-Integrated neurocognitive therapy for schizophrenic patients. Heidelberg: Springer; 2013.

Twamley. Compensatory cognitive training. 2011. www.cogsmart.com/

Relaxation Exercises

8

Relaxation techniques have been applied in psychotherapy for a long time. The ability to relax, which is acquired through exercises, has a number of positive effects for patients. These include enhanced body awareness, improved recovery from everyday stress, greater resilience in coping with acute symptoms, and increased awareness of mental processes. Further, relaxation techniques have proven valuable in therapeutic settings, especially with patients meeting CHR criteria. Relaxation exercises can offer a range of positive effects. For example:

- As with other psychiatric symptoms, there is a high correlation between the stress experienced in everyday life and the occurrence of CHR symptoms. Relaxation exercises are a suitable method for recovering from everyday stress and facing challenges in daily life more calmly. If practiced regularly, they enable patients to become more resilient to stress. However, even when used only in acute moments of stress, they can have a positive effect on the stress experienced by inducing deceleration and promoting calmness.
- Relaxation techniques play an important role in the management of CHR symptoms. On the one hand, they are suitable as coping strategies and can help to reduce or even stop acute symptoms. They can also contribute to reducing the unpleasant emotions, such as anger, anxiety, or panic, that trigger symptoms. Additionally, learning relaxation techniques can make it easier to handle a symptom. Relaxation techniques can be particularly beneficial for persistent symptoms, such as hearing voices.
- Relaxation exercises help to connect the patient with the here and now. Used correctly, they can counteract dissociative feelings that trigger many CHR symptoms. In the case of severe depersonalization, they help people to become aware of their own ego consistency: "I remain myself. Even though I feel panic right now, I am not dissolving. I am still me."
- Relaxation exercises have a positive effect on cognitive functions. They are helpful tools in moments of acute formal thinking difficulties and, when practiced frequently, can also lead to improved concentration.

N. Traber-Walker, M. Franscini, *Adolescents at Clinical High Risk for Psychosis*,
https://doi.org/10.1007/978-3-032-10341-3_8

- Relaxation exercises lead to a better understanding and recognition of certain triggers for symptoms, in the sense of taking a step back and asking oneself, "What has just happened? Why have these feelings been activated?" Recognizing the feeling behind the paranoid thought is particularly helpful with paranoid symptoms. The trigger is often some basic emotion, such as suddenly feeling afraid and believing that something is directed against the patient. If patients are able to recognize such fears as an automatic reaction to a possible trigger, rather than a real danger, they will find it easier to reflect on their thoughts.
- Practiced regularly, relaxation exercises can increase the experience of self-efficacy.

The category "Relaxation Exercises" in the worksheet "Positive Activities" describes some relaxation methods that are recommended for adolescents with CHR symptoms. Meditation techniques have deliberately not been recommended. Meditation and psychosis can be a problematic combination, as such meditative states can potentially exacerbate psychotic symptoms. Therefore, it is recommended that patients meeting CHR criteria use relaxation techniques that have a lower risk of dissociation. Relaxation techniques that involve movement, such as tai chi, qigong, yoga, Feldenkrais, or progressive muscle relaxation (PMR), have proven particularly helpful. Adolescents with CHR symptoms can also benefit from active mindfulness exercises. When starting relaxation exercises, it is useful to keep them short (10 minutes or less) and to focus on an external stimulus. Patients with dissociative symptoms, but also with panic symptoms, may find it helpful to keep their eyes open during the exercises.

Below are a number of relaxation techniques suitable for patients experiencing psychotic or CHR symptoms. Some sample exercises and instructions are also provided. The exercises should be tried out with the patient during the therapy sessions when relaxation techniques are first introduced. In this way, any unpleasant emotions that arise from the exercises can be addressed directly by the therapist. Later, patients can also practice the exercises by themselves at home. However, it is important that they have a good introduction to the techniques before they try them on their own.

Recommendations for carrying out the relaxation exercises

- It is important to adapt to the patient and to the patient's needs. Some patients prefer to sit and others to lie down. Some patients do not want to close their eyes, and this should be respected.
- Before the exercise, the therapist should explain to the patient what they are about to do, allowing the patient to prepare themselves.
- Patients can stop the exercise at any time if they feel uncomfortable.
- The exercise should be read aloud in the calmest, most monotonous voice possible.
- It is important to read aloud slowly and to pause a lot between sentences.

8.1 Mindfulness

In recent years, the term mindfulness in particular has become established. Mindfulness-based therapy methods have their roots in Eastern contemplative traditions and Buddhism. Jon Kabat-Zinn was the first to translate mindfulness-based methods for the Western world and introduce them into Western medicine and healthcare. He defines mindfulness as a particular way of bringing attention to the present moment in an intentional and non-judgmental way (Kabat-Zinn 2003). Mindfulness is primarily about awareness without changing or evaluating anything. This distinguishes mindfulness from many other relaxation exercises, as no relaxation or physical responses are consciously produced. However, non-judgmental awareness of the moment usually leads automatically to a state of relaxation.

A growing number of studies emphasize the positive influence of mindfulness exercises on physical and mental health (Bear 2003). Examples of mindfulness- and acceptance-based methods in psychotherapy include acceptance and commitment therapy (ACT) and mindfulness-based cognitive therapy (MBCT), both of which show positive effects on depression. Mindfulness is also an important component of dialectical behavioral therapy (DBT), according to Marsha Linehan, which has shown efficacy in patients with borderline personality disorder. Mindfulness- and acceptance-based methods are receiving increasing attention in psychotherapy with children and adolescents. A review by Harnett and Dawe (2012) with a total of 41 included studies showed growing evidence of a positive effect of mindfulness-based methods in children and adolescents for various psychiatric symptoms.

8.1.1 Mindful Everyday Activities

Mindfulness can be practiced very well through various basic activities. Mindful activities in everyday life remain suitable for psychotic patients or patients with severe derealization and depersonalization, as they encourage focused attention on a specific task. Thoughts are not free-floating, and the risk of dissociation is therefore low.

Patients should be encouraged to perform certain everyday activities with full concentration and awareness. Practically all daily activities are suitable for this, such as unlocking a door, brushing teeth, washing hands, preparing the bag for the next morning, or emptying the dishwasher. The aim is for patients to focus on just this one action and consciously carry out each individual, small step. During the exercise, patients should focus on their different sensory experiences. For example: “How does the key feel in my hand? How much force do I need to turn the key in the lock? Where do I feel resistance when I unlock?” This can be well practiced in therapy. Possible digression and failure of the task should be anticipated before the exercise. An important part of mindfulness is accepting digression. Patients should be told repeatedly how difficult these exercises are and that we are not used to focusing our attention so specifically on the here and now.

Instructions Example: "Write Your Name"

"Can you please write your name on a piece of paper? Please do this consciously, with your full awareness. First, place the piece of paper in front of you. Take it in your hand, hold it firmly, feel the paper between your fingers. Then consciously place it on the table in front of you. Make sure it's in the right place so you can write your name. As you place it on the table, feel your fingers release it as soon as you feel that it is placed where you would like it to be.

Now consciously pick up the pen. Remove the cap from the pen. Place the cap on the table. Exactly where you think the cap should be. Now place the pen on the paper. Start writing the first letter of your name. Then lift the pen away from the page and consciously find the place on the paper where you want to write the second letter. And so on. When you have written all the letters, pick up the lid and put it back on the pen. Now put the pen down."

Patients should be encouraged to do these mindfulness exercises as often as possible in their daily lives. Even if these exercises are difficult at first, they will become easier with practice.

8.1.2 Mindfulness Through the Five Senses

The aim of these exercises is to concentrate on a single sense and only pursue this sense, to develop awareness of each of the senses. Especially in the case of sensory illusions, these exercises can be very helpful. Patients are often unsettled by the fact that they can no longer trust their perception. This makes it all the more important to train one's own five senses. Actively experiencing, following, and feeling their own senses can be a corrective experience for patients. The exercises can also help with reality checks. What do real sounds sound like? What does it feel like to see? What does it feel like to smell? What is the sense of taste like? What tastes can be perceived? What does touch feel like? What is it like to consciously touch something?

The exercises can be done at home between appointments. It is useful to try out the exercises directly during therapy and to go through the sensory experiences together with the patient.

Many therapeutic approaches with mindfulness methods (e.g., ATC) place great emphasis on non-judgmental awareness and acceptance. This means that the mindfulness experience should not be evaluated, i.e., no questions about whether a sensation is pleasant or unpleasant. The aim is for all emotions and perceptions to be seen as subjective sensations and accepted as such. The background to this consideration is that negative emotions are just as much a part of life as positive emotions and should therefore not be avoided or suppressed. Instead, they should be accepted as a temporary feeling. The acceptance of unpleasant emotions has already been described in Chap. 5 as an important aspect of therapy. The concept of mindfulness can also be helpful here.

Patients with CHR symptoms often lose their automatic access to perceptions and have to start over in order to perceive their sensory experiences at all. This is particularly the case with derealization and depersonalization, but also with hallucinations. Therefore, it may be helpful to train sensory perception in relation to positive experiences during therapy. Patients should relearn which smells, sounds, or tactile sensations they find pleasant. Smells, for example, are often associated with memories and can trigger certain emotions. Deliberately creating certain sensory experiences can be used as a coping strategy. For example, if someone is very fond of vanilla, the smell of a vanilla pod can induce a calming, cozy feeling. The deliberate production of certain sounds can help against acoustic hallucinations. Similarly, there are pictures or colors that calm us down or cheer us up when we look at them. Conversely, aversive perceptions can trigger an unpleasant feeling and be a trigger for certain symptoms. For example, hearing a car alarm may trigger anxiety symptoms. Identifying this sound as a trigger can help patients handle the anxiety.

8.1.2.1 Sense of Taste

One exercise is to concentrate on eating or drinking something, for example, eating a piece of chocolate very slowly. Patients can also try different approaches to the same task in order to compare them. For example, eat the first piece of chocolate very quickly and the other piece very slowly and deliberately. What differences come to light between the two methods?

- How does the food feel in your mouth?
- How does it feel on your tongue?
- Where else in your body is the taste perceived?
- How long does the taste remain in your mouth after the food has been swallowed?

8.1.2.2 Sense of Touch

The sense of touch can be trained simply by touching materials. All kinds of objects are suitable, so these exercises can be done without much preparation. For example, what do the surface, edge, and underside of the table feel like? Patients can also feel their own clothes and compare the texture of the materials.

This type of exercise can be done very well in the great outdoors with stone, grass, or trees.

- What is the difference when you touch a stone, a blade of grass, or a tree?
- What stands out?
- What sensations are triggered by this?

Another way to promote tactile perception is to experiment with heat. This includes deliberately washing hands with cold or hot water or alternating showers. Another exercise can be to touch an ice cube or a warm teacup, always with intentionality and awareness.

8.1.2.3 Sense of Smell

Spices, flowers, or synthetic substances such as detergents, sunscreen, or soap are suitable for the conscious olfactory experience. Another option is to create odors, for example, by lighting a match or blowing out a candle.

- What smells do you notice?
- Where in your body do you perceive the smell?
- What physical reactions do you have to the odor?
- What does the scent make you feel?

Odors are often associated with memories and can evoke strong emotions, which makes them an effective resource. Smelling something that patients like can be a good coping strategy in difficult situations.

8.1.2.4 Conscious Listening

A lot is picked up by our hearing. Our ears are constantly taking in sound. However, there are only a few moments when our entire perception is focused on listening to these sounds. Most of the time, we hear without really listening. Awareness of listening can be practiced.

- What can you listen to?
- What sounds are you currently aware of?
- What happens when you cover your ears? Will you hear less?
- What is the difference if you close your eyes? How does that change your perception?

Conscious listening can be practiced by simply listening to sounds in the therapy office. Another possibility is to go outside and listen to all the sounds on the street, in the forest, etc. Without access to the outdoors, music can be a good method, for example, by consciously listening to a piece of music and trying to concentrate only on the instrumentation.

8.1.2.5 Sense of Sight

Conscious awareness of sight can be a particularly helpful exercise for patients with hallucinations and illusions. Visual awareness exercises may help patients become more aware of the differences between real images and hallucinations, and conscious awareness of what is seen can be a helpful grounding technique for dissociative symptoms. Since visual awareness can be practiced at any time and in any place, it is useful in its versatility. When first introduced to this type of mindful activity, patients should be asked to consciously look at a scene, a picture, or an object.

- What do you see in front of you?
- What does this image section look like?
- What colors do you see?
- What kind of shapes?

8.1.3 Mindful Walking

Walking meditation is a good way of focusing on the present moment. People walk over and over again, almost casually. Walking happens mostly unconsciously. Becoming aware of the process of walking can help develop mindfulness out of automatic processes. In addition, mindful walking can help to calm patients in stressful moments, regardless of which symptoms are most prominent. The exercise can be done anytime, anywhere.

Patients can be encouraged to walk at varying speeds—either quickly or very slowly—while becoming aware of each individual step. Mindful walking reveals how much is required to take a single step and which parts of the body and their muscles are used when walking.

8.1.4 Observe the Breath

The aim of conscious breathing exercises is to observe one's own breathing for a short period of time. Patients should try to concentrate only on their breathing. It is important that they do not try to change, direct, or control their breathing. They should simply observe their breath as it is. It is best to practice this in an upright sitting position, as this reduces the risk of dissociation compared to lying down. Patients with severe dissociation or anxiety symptoms are also advised not to close their eyes during this exercise, as keeping the eyes open helps them to stay more grounded in the present moment and minimizes the risk of experiencing perceived threats. In more stable phases of therapy, when patients have practiced these exercises several times and are not experiencing acute symptoms, closing the eyes may be beneficial. This approach encourages facing and enduring possible feelings of panic, rather than avoiding them.

Instructions for Observing the Breathing

"Take a few minutes for yourself. Make sure that for the next few minutes you are not disturbed, i.e., *you are not distracted by external stimuli. The aim is for you to observe your breath as such for the next few minutes. Sit in a comfortable position with your feet firmly on the floor and your arms resting on your lap, a table, or the back of a chair. You can keep your eyes open or close them if you prefer. Watch your breathing for the next few minutes. Continue to breathe as before. You should not change or control your breathing. It's not about breathing faster or slower or deeper. Just try to be aware of how you are breathing. Breathe in and breathe out. Then in and out again. And so on. Try to do this for the next twenty breaths.*

It doesn't matter if your attention wanders; that's normal. You don't need to push away your wandering thoughts; just acknowledge that they are there. Then gently bring your attention back to your breath. Breathe in, breathe out, breathe in, breathe out..."

There are several variations of this exercise. Patients can also be instructed to breathe in a specific way, for example, first breathing into the chest and then into the abdomen, allowing them to compare the differences between the two types of breathing.

An alternative option is to count the breaths and try to inhale and exhale for exactly the same amount of time. Here, patients can be guided to lengthen their breaths, inhaling and exhaling twice as long as before.

Another exercise is to observe the differences in the exercise when sitting, standing, and lying down. What do they notice or feel differently in each position?

The aim of these breathing exercises is to teach patients how to relax in a short time and find their way back to themselves in moments of stress. These exercises are very simple and can be done anywhere, for example, on the bus or while waiting.

8.1.5 Body Scan

This exercise is based on the methods of Jon Kabat-Zinn. The body scan is designed to help you focus your attention on specific areas of the body and notice how those parts of the body feel. First, attention is directed to different parts of the body, one after the other. For example, starting with the left foot, the focus then gradually moves up the leg to the hip, then to the other leg, and finally up the entire body to the head. At the end, attention is brought to the whole body. If the attention wanders during the exercise, it should be registered without judgment, and the focus can be gently returned to the body.

Body Scan Instructions

"First, take five deep breaths, in and out. Try to focus on your breath and let your thoughts pass by. Thoughts will come up throughout the exercise and may distract you. Simply acknowledge the thought, recognize it, and try to let it go. Aim to focus your attention on the exercise and stay present in the here and now.

Start by focusing your attention on your right foot. Try to feel your foot as fully as possible. Feel each toe individually. Start with your big toe, then move to your index toe, your middle toe, your fourth toe, and then your little toe. Feel each toe separately. What sensations do you notice? Now move your attention to the ball of your right foot. How does it feel? What sensations do you notice? Try to concentrate fully on the ball of your right foot.

Now move your focus to your right heel. How does your heel feel? And feel the sensations of your entire right foot.

Slowly move your attention to your right lower leg. What do you feel here? Then focus on your right knee. What sensations do you register there?

Now focus on your right thigh. What sensations are there in your right thigh? Focus all your attention on your right thigh.

Now focus your attention on your whole right leg, including your right foot. What are you feeling there? Notice all the sensations in your body without judgment. Just notice them.

Now move your attention to your left foot. Feel your left big toe. How does it feel? Now the left second toe. How does the second toe feel? And the middle toe, can you feel it? Can you feel your fourth toe? Now your little toe, how does it feel? Your toes on your left foot, how do they feel? Focus your attention on that.

Now move your attention to the ball of your left foot. What sensations do you feel? How does it feel? Your heel, your left heel. Focus all your attention on your left heel.

Now your whole left foot. How does it rest? What do you notice? Do you notice any difference from before? How does your left foot feel?

Now move your attention to your left lower leg. Your left lower leg, how does it feel? What do you notice?

And move up to your left knee. Can you feel your left knee? What do you notice?

Your left thigh, how does it feel? What do you feel?

Now focus your attention on your whole left leg and your left foot. What are you feeling there?

Now focus your attention on each of your two legs. What do you feel? Follow your sensations.

Move your attention to the right side of your bottom, and focus on how it feels.

Now move your attention to the left side of your bottom. What do you feel? What does your left bottom feel like?

Now bring your attention into your abdomen. Allow your full attention to rest in your belly for a moment. What are you feeling in your belly?

Next bring your attention to the chest area. Focus on how your chest feels. What sensations are you experiencing here?

Now focus your attention on your lower back. What are you feeling? What does your lower back feel like?

Gently continue to move your attention up along your spine. Bring your attention to your upper back. How does it feel?

Then move your attention to your right shoulder. How does it feel? What does your right shoulder feel like?

Continue along your right arm. First your upper arm. What do you feel?

Now move your attention to your right elbow. Feel the sensations in your right elbow.

Next, try to focus all your attention on your right hand. The back of your hand. Your fingers. Your thumb—feel your thumb. Now focus all your attention on your right index finger. Then your right middle finger. What do you feel?

Now focus your attention on your right ring finger. Then focus all your attention on your smallest right finger. Now feel your whole right hand.

And focus all your attention on your right arm and hand. What do you feel? What do your right arm and your right hand feel like?

Now focus all your attention on your left shoulder. What does your left shoulder feel like? Focus all your attention on your left shoulder.

Switch your attention to your left upper arm. What does your left upper arm feel like?

Your left elbow; focus all your attention on your left elbow. Now your left forearm, what do you feel there?

Then your left hand. Engage with the feelings in your left hand. Your fingers. First your left thumb. What does your left thumb feel like? Now your left forefinger, what do you feel there?

Now your left middle finger, what do you feel there? What do you notice?

Can you feel the index finger of your left hand? And focus on your left little finger.

8.2 Progressive Muscle Relaxation (PMR)

Progressive muscle relaxation (PMR) was developed by Dr. Edmund Jacobson in the USA at the end of the 1930s. The principle of the method is to first tense and then release the tension within a set muscle group, which automatically induces relaxation.

This exercise promotes relaxation at any time and augments awareness of one's own body. Regular practice promotes greater calm, serenity and balance, and improves concentration. It can also help to relieve muscular tension and sleep problems.

It is very popular with young patients. Even patients who otherwise find it difficult to engage in relaxation exercises are often interested in PMR. Since it seems less esoteric and suspicious than other relaxation exercises, and the risk of loss of control or even dissociation is very low, PMR is particularly suitable for patients with symptoms of derealization and depersonalization. The exercises help release constant tension and allow patients to feel and consciously direct individual parts of the body.

While the PMR instructions described below take about 15 minutes to complete and involve almost every muscle in the body, it is possible to use shorter PMR exercises in everyday life. An additional option is to tense and relax one part of the body at a time, for example, making a fist and letting go. The exercise can be repeated as often as necessary until the effect is achieved. The 'spaghetti' exercise, which is recommended for several symptoms in the symptom management chapter, is a further option. It involves contracting and relaxing all sorts of muscles at once. The exercises can be done in any situation, unnoticed by others. As a result, these techniques can also be used to treat anxiety, increased irritability, and impulsivity.

Instructions for Progressive Muscle Relaxation

Tighten your right fist and hold it for one or two breaths.

Now release. Repeat this once more.

Now make a fist with your left hand and hold it. Breathe deeply in and out, in and out. Now release. Make a fist with your left hand again. Make it very tight. Breathe in, breathe out, breathe in, breathe out. Let go now. Feel it. Feel the difference from before.

Now tense your right arm. As hard as you can. Very tense, all the muscles. Breathe in, breathe out. Release again. Tense again. Very hard. Even harder, all the muscles. Breathe in deeply and breathe out. Now let go. Feel it. Relax, how does your right arm feel?

Next, tense all the muscles in your left arm. As hard as you can. Breathe in, breathe out. Breathe in, breathe out. Now let go. Feel for yourself. What does your left arm feel like? Is it different from the right? Tense your left arm again. As much as you can, flex all your muscles. Breathe in deeply, breathe out deeply. Now let go. Notice how your left arm feels.

At the same time, pull your shoulder blades up and back. Breathe in, breathe out. Now let it go. Let them fall. Pull them back up, very firmly. Tense them towards the spine. Breathe in and out. Now let go.

Pull your chest together. As hard as you can. Now breathe into your chest, very shallowly. Now let go. Feel it. Breathe in and out deeply.

And again: tense your whole chest. Breathe in and out briefly. Now let go again. Breathe in and out deeply and feel. How does your chest feel?

Next tense all your abdominal muscles. Very tightly. And breathe in and out of your chest. Now let go of your stomach muscles. Feel your belly; breathe deeply, in and out, into your belly. Now tense all your abdominal muscles again, as hard as you can. Now let go again. Feel it.

Now squeeze your glutes as hard as you can. Hold this for two breaths. Breathe in and out, in and out. That's good. Now let go. Feel for yourself. Breathe in and out. Squeeze your glutes again. As hard as you can. Breathe in and out. Now let go. Let everything go.

Next, tense your right leg. Tense all the muscles in your right leg as hard as you can. Very tense. Breathe deeply in and out. In and out. Now let go. Breathe through. Feel your right leg. Now tense it again. Tense all the muscles in your right leg as much as you can. Breathe in and out. And again. Breathe in and out. Then let go. Let all the muscles go. Breathe in and out. How do you feel? How does your right leg feel?

Now tense your left leg. Tense all the muscles in your left leg. As hard as you can. Breathe in and out. Breathe in and out. Let go. Release your left leg. Breathe in and out; feel it. Tense your left leg again. Tense all the muscles in your left leg as much as you can. Breathe in and out deeply. Breathe in and out again. Now let go. Let everything go. Feel your left leg. Tense your right foot and curl your toes. Squeeze as hard as you can. Breathe in and out. Breathe in and out. Then let go. Feel it. How does your foot feel? Take a deep breath. Now tense your right foot again and tense all your toes. As hard as you can. Breathe in and out. Breathe in and out. Then let go. Feel it. What does your right foot feel like?

Tense your left foot. Roll your toes together and tense your foot as much as you can. Breathe in and out. Breathe in and out. Now let go. Release your left foot. Squeeze it again, including the toes. Breathe deeply, in and out. Now let go.

Next, tense your face. Tense your facial muscles. Press your lips together, narrow your eyes, and wrinkle your forehead. Now let it all go again. And feel it. Now try again, tensing all your facial muscles as hard as you can. Keep them tensed. Then let go again.

Now try to tense all the muscles in your body, from head to toe, as hard as you can. Very tense. Breathe in deeply again, holding the tension, and breathe out.

Now, as you breathe out, release all the tension at once. Relax every muscle in your body. Breathe in and out slowly and naturally, feeling the relaxation.

Then begin to tense all your muscles again, from head to toe, tense them as much as you can. Breathe in and out. Breathe in and out. Now let go. Let everything go. Let go of all the tension and let go of the muscles in your body, and feel the effect.

Further Reading

Bear RA. Mindfulness training as a clinical intervention: a conceptual and empirical review. Clin Psychol Sci Pract. 2003;10:12–143.

Harnett PH, Dawe S. Review: the contribution of mindfulness-based therapies for children and families and proposed conceptual integration. Child Adolesc Mental Health. 2012;17:95–208.

Hayes SC. Acceptance and mindfulness treatment for children & adolescents: a practitioner's guide. Oakland: The New Harbinger Publications Inc.; 2008.

Hayes SC, Follette VM, Linehan MM. Mindfulness and acceptance. Expanding the cognitive-behavioural tradition. New York: Gilford; 2004.

Hölzel BK, Lazar SW, Gard T, Schuman-Oliver ZS, Vago DR, Ott U. How does mindfulness mediation work? Proposing mechanism of action from a conceptual and neural perspective. Perspect Psychol Sci. 2011;6(6):537–59.

Kabat-Zinn J. Mindfulness-based interventions in context: past, present, and future. Clin Psychol Sci Pract. 2003;10:144–56.

Shonin E, Van Gordon W, Griffiths MD. Do mindfulness-based therapies have a role in the treatment of psychosis? Aust N Z J Psychiatry. 2014; https://doi.org/10.1177/0004867413512688.

9 Resource Management

Improving self-esteem and self-efficacy is one of the most important aspects of any psychotherapy. Particularly with adolescents meeting CHR criteria, a lot of time should be invested in this work. Many adolescent patients have been struggling with self-esteem issues pre-morbidly, and the new, often frightening symptoms make them feel even more insecure. There may also be experiences of failure as a result of the symptoms, such as a decline in school performance, conflicts with peers, or a decline in physical performance.

Strengthening existing resources and focusing on small successes in everyday life can be very helpful.

Several studies have also shown that patients, particularly those with severe psychiatric symptoms, respond positively to solution-focused strategies in therapy. They prefer to have more positive content in their sessions rather than focusing on pathological aspects.

Solution-focused therapy begins with the attitude of the therapist. It is important that the therapist believes that the patient is capable of change. Although many adolescents who come to counseling are severely affected by their symptoms and the symptoms take up a lot of space in their daily lives, it is important to be aware of the healthy aspects of the person. It is the healthy parts of the patient that motivate them to come to therapy. However, when adolescents come to therapy at the request of their parents and are only moderately motivated, focusing on the positive constructs can be very effective. In fact, oppositional, unmotivated adolescents cooperate surprisingly well when therapy consists mainly of discussing their strengths and activities they enjoy.

Supplementary Information The online version contains supplementary material available at https://doi.org/10.1007/978-3-032-10341-3_9. The videos can be accessed individually by clicking the DOI link in the accompanying figure caption or by scanning this link with the SN More Media App.

N. Traber-Walker, M. Franscini, *Adolescents at Clinical High Risk for Psychosis*,
https://doi.org/10.1007/978-3-032-10341-3_9

Resources such as hobbies, special talents, and helpful social relationships should be explored during the diagnostic phase. As mentioned in the chapter on family counseling, parents should also be asked about their child's strengths. Positive statements from third parties about the patient should be shared with them.

As a therapist, it is helpful to make a note of the patient's resources during the initial contact and to write down the positive things that are noticed.

9.1 Who Am I?

Finding one's own identity is one of the most important but also most difficult developmental tasks during adolescence. Especially at the onset of CHR symptoms, many adolescents experience a major change in their personality and are confused by it. Symptoms such as hallucinations, depersonalization, derealization, and paranoid ideation are particularly destabilizing.

Establishing one's own identity is also an important topic in therapy. The therapist should explore how the young patients see themselves. Who are they and who do they want to become? What are their values? What are their strengths? What personal qualities are important to them? When working with CHR patients, it has proven helpful for them to create collages or pictures that represent their personality. See the worksheet "Who Am I?"

9.2 Working with Names

The aim of the exercise is to write the patient's first name vertically on a sheet of paper and find a word for each letter that suits the young person. The therapist should ensure that the words are generally positive or neutral. Patients may find this task difficult at first, but they generally enjoy it.

Name: Michael

M: motivated
I: interested
C: cool style
H: honest
A: Amsterdam
E: enthusiastic
L: likes to laugh

Therapeutic Conversation with Michael

Michael:	Hm, M... no idea. I used to be motivated and good at motivating others.
Therapist:	Not anymore?
Michael:	Well, I'm often tired and have no energy, so the opposite: lack of motivation.
Therapist:	And there are no more situations where you are motivated or motivate others?
Michael:	Sometimes there are.
Therapist:	Has there been such a situation recently?
Michael:	(thinking) At the weekend. I went out with four friends. We wanted to go to a party, but then everyone got tired and a bit lazy. I insisted that we should just go by, and if we didn't like the party, we could leave soon. So I motivated everyone. It was a great night. After the party, my friends said that they were glad I had insisted on going.
Therapist:	So is it fair to say that motivation is a quality that defines you?
Michael:	Yes, it is.
Therapist:	Next letter: I. What does "I" make you think of?
Michael:	I'm interested in many things.
Michael:	C? Difficult ... My friends would say that I have a cool style.
Therapist:	Do you think so?
Michael:	Well ... actually yes.
Michael:	H... maybe honest.
Therapist:	Are you an honest person?
Michael:	Yeah, I think so. More than others, I think. But I lie sometimes.
Therapist:	Who doesn't?
Michael:	(laughs)
Therapist:	But in general, you're an honest person.
Michael:	I'm honest, yes.
Michael:	A ... Amsterdam? My grandmother is from Holland. And it's my favorite city.
Therapist:	Okay, then Amsterdam. The next letter is E.
Michael:	I would say enthusiastic. It's something that suits me very well.
Therapist:	Yes, I've noticed that too.
Therapist:	That leaves the L.
Michael:	L ... I like to laugh.

9.3 Video Messages

All therapists are probably familiar with this: There are sessions when patients seem to be doing very well and have little interest in talking about difficulties. Instead of focusing on a possible future change for the worse, these sessions can be used to develop prevention strategies for the next crisis. It is important for patients to keep reminding themselves that change does happen and that there are always good moments.

One method that has proved successful in clinical practice is working with video messages. Patients are videotaped during the session. They talk about how they feel and what helped them feel so good today. They give themselves advice for more difficult times. The videos can be recorded; ideally, patients agree to record them on their mobile phones. This gives them the opportunity to watch the video again and again without being venue-dependent.

It is also useful for the therapist to have a version of the video. If the patient is in a bad mood in a later session, the video can be watched together. In difficult moments, young people are often hesitant to watch these videos because they feel uncomfortable watching themselves. However, once they are involved, they usually feel a sense of relief. They automatically become more relaxed, and they often smile. In our experience, watching the video together makes the young people feel more confident and generally more active.

Alternatively, instead of a video message, patients can write a letter of advice to themselves.

9.4 Media Libraries

Media of all kinds can be a wonderful resource when it comes to boosting mood or activating drive. Normally, people feel good when they look at holiday photos or photos of their loved ones. Most people also have songs that motivate, energize, or cheer them up.

However, many patients find it overwhelming to search for photos or download songs when they are feeling down. Creating media libraries for bad moments has been shown to be effective. These can include photo libraries of holiday memories, pictures of important people, favorite animals, idols, or even places in the world they would like to visit. It is useful to create such a library on their mobile phone, where they can access it at any time. An analog photo book of favorite pictures compiled by the patient can also be very useful. Music playlists for all moods are also recommended, preferably on the mobile phone. A collection of mantras and quotes is also very helpful for many young people. These can be quotes from stars or song lyrics chosen by the adolescent.

Patients should have a free choice in the creation of the libraries. It is not up to us as therapists to judge which pictures, songs, or mantras are appropriate. It makes more sense to take an interest in why the person idolizes a particular person or finds a particular photo helpful. Idols and role models can be included in therapy.

9.5 List of Strengths

Most patients initially have difficulty naming their strengths. When asked about their strengths, they will often say that they don't know or that they don't have any. As a therapist, it is important not to be discouraged by such statements but to continue exploring until the patient has come up with at least five strengths.

Helpful questions can be:

- What are you good at?
- What do you like best about yourself?
- What school subjects are you strongest in?
- What is a quality you don't want to lose?

- Why do your friends like you?
- What would your mother/father/sister, etc., say?
- What do you get compliments for?

Each answer should be immediately followed by the question “What else?“to encourage them to think of more strengths.

In the end, most adolescents are surprised at how many strengths they were able to identify during the discussion.

List of Strengths

Having a list of personal strengths in the app gives patients an easily accessible reminder of their abilities, helping to build their confidence and resilience. Whenever they feel uncertain or face challenges, they can refer to the list to remind them of their strengths and help them feel more empowered.

Further explanations on working with the Robin Z app’s strength list in the therapy session can be found in the tutorial video “**Library**” (Fig. 9.1).

In the Robin View evaluation program (tutorial video “Robin View”), the Robin Z-strength list of patients is displayed graphically (Fig. 9.2).

Information on how the data is sent to Robin View can be found in the tutorial video “**Share My Data**” (Fig. 9.3).

Therapeutic Conversation with Lucy

Therapist:	You have no strengths at all? That can’t be right. Think about it carefully.
Lucy:	(shakes her head) I can’t think of anything at the moment.
Therapist:	Well, I know a few things. But I think you have to work them out for yourself. There’s no point in me listing your strengths.
Lucy:	But I don’t know any strengths.
Therapist:	That’s not true. Think about it: What are you really good at? Better than others?
Lucy:	Well, maybe dancing. At least I used to. Now I don’t go to practice as regularly.
Therapist:	So dancing. First strength to write down. And what is important in dancing?
Lucy:	(thinks for a moment) well, you should have coordination and a feeling for the music.
Therapist:	Do you have both?
Lucy:	I think so.
Therapist:	So that’s two more strengths. What else?
Lucy:	I’m actually quite sporty. I’m very good at sports at school.
Therapist:	Sporty then. What else?
Lucy:	I’m also good at languages. At least German and English.
Therapist:	Are there any other subjects you are good at?

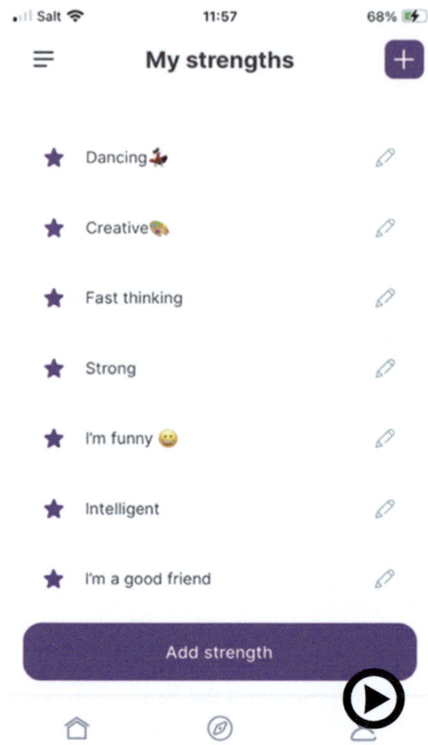

Fig. 9.1 Tutorial video "Library" (▶ https://doi.org/10.1007/000-k5q)

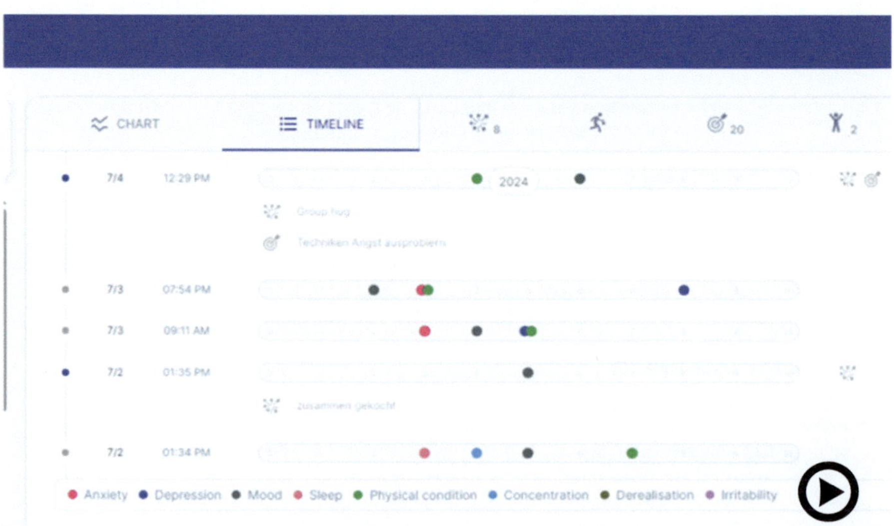

Fig. 9.2 Tutorial video "Robin View" (▶ https://doi.org/10.1007/000-k5p)

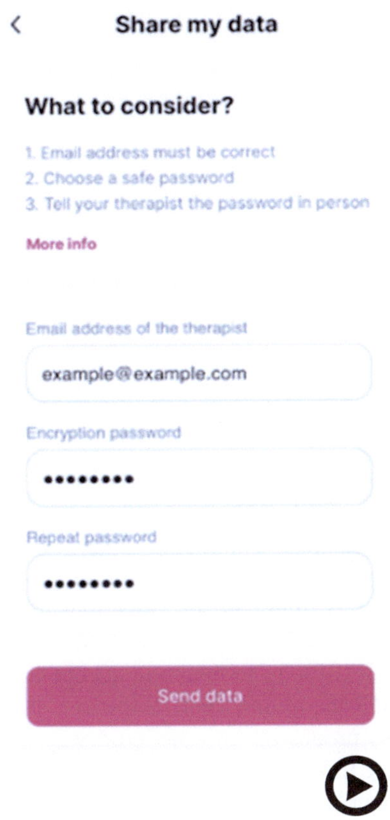

Fig. 9.3 Tutorial video "Share my data" (▶ https://doi.org/10.1007/000-k5n)

Lucy:	History. And chemistry.
Therapist:	Wow, that's quite a lot. Considering you said you weren't good at anything. (Lucy laughs a little.)
Therapist:	Wow, language, dancing, and sports. Could it be that you are very creative?
Lucy:	I don't know, maybe. My mum says that sometimes, yeah.
Therapist:	See, if even your mum says it, how does your mum know?
Lucy:	Because I'm good at drawing. Or sometimes I make beautiful table decorations and arrange my room nicely.
Therapist:	So you're good at decorating and drawing, too?
Lucy:	(shrugs her shoulders) A little. But other people can do it too, like my dad.
Therapist:	Strengths do not mean that you are the only person who is good at it. Of course, there are other people who are good at decorating, drawing, or dancing. But you're still good at it. That doesn't mean you're the best or most talented dancer. We're not looking for your extraordinary talent; we're looking for the things you're good at and that you like about yourself. And we've already found a few things. What else do you like about yourself? What character traits?

Lucy:	(thinks for a moment) I try to be nice. To help others.
Therapist:	So Nice and helpful? Nice is a very general word. What exactly do you mean by being nice?
Lucy:	I am friendly to others. I can empathize well with others. I am polite.
Therapist:	So friendly, empathetic, and polite. What else?
Lucy:	I am there for others, and I am a good listener.
Therapist:	(nods) go on?
Lucy:	I can make people laugh.
Therapist:	So you're funny? That's very important. Making people laugh is a great quality. There are lots of people who can't do that at all. You know, for someone who has no strengths at all, you sure have compiled quite a long list.
Lucy:	(laughs) that's true. I never thought I'd come up with so much. It wasn't even that difficult.

9.6 List of Compliments

Like the list of strengths, the list of compliments is about making patients aware of their resources and positive qualities. Most people are sensitive to negative criticism and easily remember what bad comments others have made about them. Compliments, on the other hand, are usually forgotten rather quickly. Especially in times of emotional distress, people tend to remember only failures and negative feedback.

Many adolescents find it difficult to hear and accept compliments. This can be further exacerbated by CHR symptoms such as distrust. Positive feedback is often questioned and sometimes processed in a paranoid way. In therapy, the focus on positive feedback should be trained so that compliments are more easily recognized and accepted. The worksheet "List of Compliments" is used to collect positive feedback. It is recommended to give the list to the patients and ask them to collect compliments over a week. Thereby, additional strengths can be noticed and added to the list of strengths.

Our observation in clinical practice is that none of the patients return to the next session with an empty list. Indeed, most patients realize that they receive more compliments in everyday life than they would have expected.

Therapeutic Conversation with Lucy

Therapist:	Have you continued your list of compliments?
Lucy:	*(shows her)*
Therapist:	And there are so many different types of compliments. You've been complimented on your looks, like you have pretty hair or a good style. Then you have been complimented on your talent for dancing. And also a lot of nice compliments about your character.
Lucy:	Well, what you said is true. If I pay attention, I notice that I get compliments almost every day.
Therapist:	How do you feel when you look at this list?
Lucy:	It makes me very happy, of course. But at the same time, I don't know. Somehow, when I look at the list, it doesn't seem real.

Therapist:	What do you mean by that?
Lucy:	I'm not sure if they're serious.
Therapist:	What makes you think that?
Lucy:	I wonder if the others at school often say nice things but make fun of me afterwards. They say, "you're so pretty," and then laugh behind my back because I believed them.
Therapist:	Do you have any evidence to support this hypothesis?
Lucy:	My friend Anna said to me on Monday, "you look so pretty today." after she said it, she looked at Leo, and he smiled at her.
Therapist:	Did Leo hear what Anna said to you?
Lucy:	I don't think so; he was too far away to hear it. But maybe she told him beforehand that she was going to say that to me.
Therapist:	Is there another explanation?
Lucy:	Hm, I think Leo really likes Anna. Maybe that's why he smiled at her.
Therapist:	Which of the two explanations do you think is more likely?
Lucy:	I think it's 50/50 for both.
Therapist:	Okay, you think both are equally likely. If we assume the first version is true, how do you feel about that?
Lucy:	Of course, I'm not feeling great. I feel ridiculed, unwanted, and sad.
Therapist:	But if you consider that Anna meant her compliment seriously and that Leo's smile had nothing to do with it?
Lucy:	Sure, I feel better.
Therapist:	If we look at the other compliments on the list, there are quite a few. And you have received many compliments several times from different people. What are the chances that none of these compliments are meant seriously?
Lucy:	Well, some of them are probably true. I just don't know which ones.
Therapist:	So does it make sense to doubt all compliments? Does it do any good?
Lucy:	No, not really. It just makes me feel worse when I think about which compliments are not meant seriously.

9.7 Look for Own Resources

The worksheet "My Resources Portfolio" is intended to help patients create a positive image of themselves that they can build on in difficult situations.

It is divided into four parts:

- Feet and legs as a foundation: The foundation should be based on what has already been achieved. A collection of everything the patient has achieved so far includes every success, no matter how small.
- The belly: The center represents gut feeling and inner peace. Helpful thoughts or guiding mantras that encourage the patient to carry on in difficult moments should be noted.
- Arms and hands: We work with our arms and hands. They represent strength and resources. The patient's strengths are noted in the arms and include personal talents and positive character traits on which they can rely.
- The crown: The crown represents the best, i.e., things that evoke particular pride for the patient. These can be character traits or achievements and may be items repeated in previous categories or entirely new.

The fifth item on the worksheet is the environment. In addition to the resources listed in the above process, loved ones such as family or friends can be listed. Activities that make the person feel good, such as hobbies or special interests, can also be recorded. Some of these things are dependent on conditions that are outside the person's control. They are therefore external to the person. They should therefore be noted around the figure itself. Only things that are independent of the environment and that the patient can rely on should be included in the figure. No one can take away past successes, talents, or character traits, no matter how difficult the current life situation. Even if a musically gifted person no longer finds the motivation or time to play the piano, the talent for music remains.

Therapeutic Conversation with Michael

Therapist:	Let's start with your legs in this worksheet. What are your achievements? What have you achieved so far that you are proud of?
Michael:	Not really anything at all.
Therapist:	Really? That surprises me. Have you never done anything well?
Michael:	Well, maybe that I've found my apprenticeship.
Therapist:	Yes, exactly. It wasn't that easy. You can be really proud of that.
Michael:	(smiles) that's right, I did beat all the other applicants.
Therapist:	Not only did you find an apprenticeship. You also passed your probationary period.
Michael:	(nods and writes it down)
Therapist:	But before you started your apprenticeship, you had to finish school.
Michael:	Well, my last diploma wasn't exactly brilliant.
Therapist:	After all, you have a high school diploma. Not everyone can say that.
Michael:	That's true. And I was really good at French.
Therapist:	Ha, that's two new points: Completed secondary school and learned French.
Michael:	I worked really hard in the first semester of my apprenticeship. I got really good grades.
Therapist:	Well, write that down. What else? What else did you do well?
Michael:	Hm, I don't know. I didn't have that many successes.
Therapist:	What happened in football? You were really good there.
Michael:	That's right. Before I gave it up because it was too much with my vocational training, I had a really good season. I scored the winning goals in several games. I even got my team promoted to a higher league.
Therapist:	Wow, that's really something. Then there was the party you told me about the other week. Where you played music?
Michael:	(starts glowing): Exactly, it was a really great feeling. People were so enthusiastic.
Therapist:	That really is a lot of success. What else?
Michael:	I once organized this fundraising marathon at school with two friends. It was for refugee aid. We raised a lot of money. I think that counts as a success, doesn't it?
Therapist:	(nods) that is really a great achievement. And what about those two friends? Are you still friends with them?
Michael:	Yes, of course. We've known each other since kindergarten. They're both my best friends. Although we don't have much contact these days.
Therapist:	Since kindergarten. That is a long time. It's not at all a matter of course to have such long-lasting friendships. Not everyone has that. Have you had any other successes?
Michael:	I think that's it for now.

Therapist:	Who knows, maybe you'll think of something later. Do you have a personal slogan? A life quote? A statement that suits you and gives you courage?
Michael:	Hm, not really. But a friend of mine posted something good on Instagram today. The sun comes up every day. I think that's pretty good.
Therapist:	Great. Then why don't you write that in the belly area? Another phrase? A saying that gives you courage?
Michael:	It's a cliché, but I like carpe diem.
Therapist nods:	Yes, that's a good one too. Now your strengths. Write your strengths on your arms. We already have quite a few that we collected with your name. Do you remember them?
Michael:	(thinks for a moment) M was motivational, H for honest, L for laughing, C for cool, I for interested, and E for enthusiastic. What was A again? Oh yes, Amsterdam. That's not a strong point now.
Therapist:	But do you like to travel and discover new cities? Widen your horizons?
Michael:	I'm open.
Therapist:	And next? What would your friends say?
Michael:	(laughs) I'm a good party person. But I'm also good at talking and listening.
Therapist:	That is a very important quality. A lot of people can't do that.
Therapist:	Now for your crown. What would you say are the five best things about you?
Michael:	I would say my openness, that I have a lot of ideas, and that I am sporty.
Therapist:	Two more to go. What else?
Michael:	That I get on well with a lot of people.
Therapist:	So popular?
Michael:	(hesitates) A silly word. But it's true.
Therapist:	Well, the last one. What else should be added to your crown?
Michael:	(thinks for a while and then says) that I never gave up, no matter how bad things got for me.
Therapist:	Very good. Now look at the page. How does it make you feel?
Michael:	Wow. It feels really good.
Therapist:	And it's all just you. No one else has anything to do with these resources. You have already achieved your successes, which no one can ever take away from you. No matter what else happens. And here are all your strengths to build on.
Michael:	I never thought I knew so many positive things about myself.

9.8 Positive Experiences

The aim here is to record the little magic moments in everyday life. Therefore, patients are encouraged to write down positive experiences on the worksheet "Positive Experiences." Especially in difficult times, people tend to have tunnel vision and lose sight of the positive. In addition, many people with CHR symptoms actually experience failure in many areas of daily life and are therefore often confronted with disappointment. This makes it all the more important for them to focus on the good parts of their lives.

Focusing on small successes and everyday pleasures can make a big difference. This does not always have to be passing the high school qualification exam; it can be getting a good grade on a difficult exam or simply the fact that the patient has managed to focus on something for an hour despite having difficulty concentrating.

More attention should be given to small things that bring joy in everyday life. These are things like when parents cook a favorite meal or the release of a favorite TV series. They may include events like receiving a like on their Instagram photo or an old friend being in touch for a long time. It is helpful to collect the events of the current day during the therapy session to give patients ideas of what they could pay attention to.

The clinical experience is that over time, the young people become increasingly successful in paying attention to such positive events. Patients find this type of protocol helpful and are happy to present their lists after the week.

Positive Experiences

The patients can use the app to record their positive experiences. This has the advantage that the experiences can be recorded immediately after they happen, making them easier to capture and remember. They can also write down their positive experiences in the logbook, so there is an opportunity to reflect on what went well in a given day when completing the logs.

The collection of positive moments can be revisited during difficult times, helping to lift the patient's spirits and reinforce the positive aspects of their lives.

Further information on therapeutic work with positive experiences can be found in the tutorial video "**Library**" (Fig. 9.4).

Therapeutic Conversation with Lucy

Lucy:	Nothing good has happened today. Nothing at all.
Therapist:	Then let's go through the day. How did you get up? What happened this morning?
Lucy:	Terrible. I slept far too little, woke up too late, and had a headache. I didn't even have time for a shower. Everything had to be done very quickly. Then I almost missed the tram and was out of breath on the tram. Of course, there was no free seat, so I had to stand.
Therapist:	But you caught the tram, you didn't miss it.
Lucy:	Yes, fortunately.
Therapist:	What were you doing on the tram?
Lucy:	Nothing. Listening to music.
Therapist:	Listening to music is nothing?
Lucy:	*(has to smile)* yes, no. it still wasn't good.

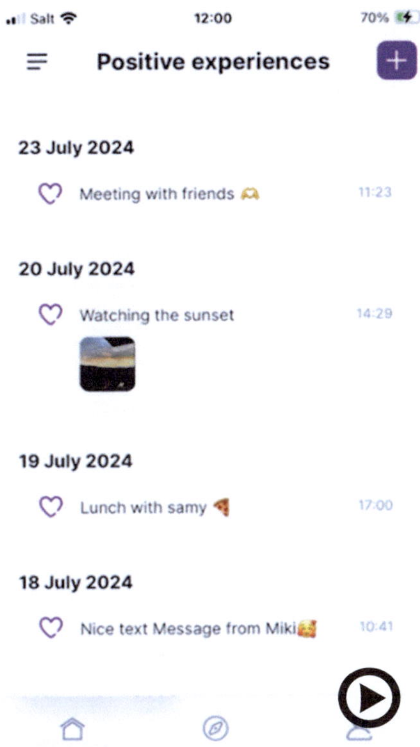

Fig. 9.4 Tutorial video "Library" (▶ https://doi.org/10.1007/000-k5r)

Therapist:	What happened then? You went to school?
Lucy:	Yes, but I was already completely exhausted when I got there.
Therapist:	At least you went. Despite little sleep, headaches, and stress.
Lucy:	I've been absent so often; I knew I had to. Otherwise, there'd be even more stress.
Therapist:	I still think it's great that you managed to go to school. Many people wouldn't be able to do that if they were you.
Lucy:	Hm.
Therapist:	How did your day go? Was school exciting?
Lucy:	Not at all. And I couldn't concentrate either.
Therapist:	How was the 10 o'clock break?
Lucy:	Normal. I was outside with my friends.
Therapist:	So, was that good?
Lucy:	Well. Yes. It was pretty funny. We laughed a lot, so that was a good moment.
Therapist:	Then you can write it down.

9.9 Worksheets

The following worksheets (Fig. 9.5) belong to this chapter and are available online for download in the context of the electronic chapter:

- Worksheet 48 “Who am I?”
- Worksheet 49 “My Strengths”.
- Worksheet 50 “List of Compliments“.
- Worksheet 51 “My Resources Portfolio”.
- Worksheet 52 “Positive Experiences”.

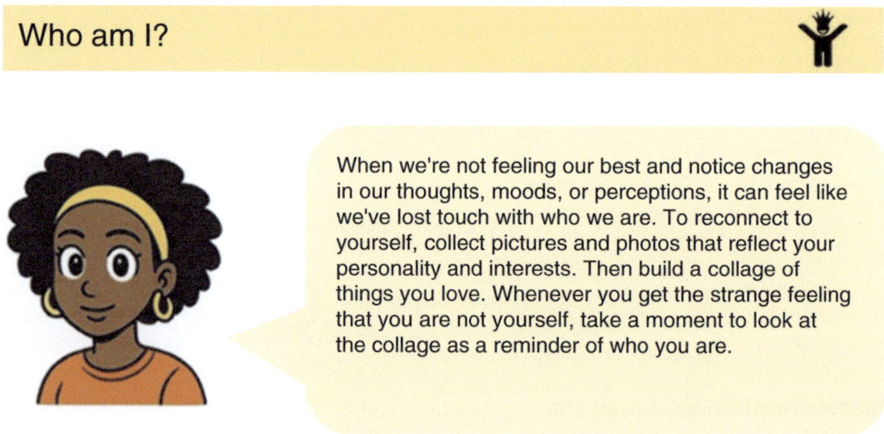

Fig. 9.5 Worksheet 48 to Worksheet 52

My Strengths

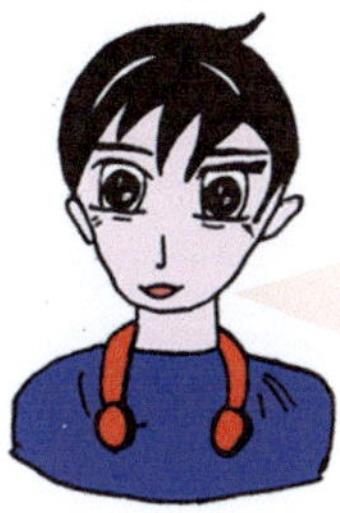

What do you like about yourself, and what aspects would you never want to change? What do people like about you? What do people often compliment you on? We all have our strengths, qualities and skills that make us who we are and that we can really value in ourselves.
In challenging times, it's especially important to recognise and focus on these strengths, as they can provide valuable resources for overcoming difficulties.

Fig. 9.5 (continued)

List of Compliments

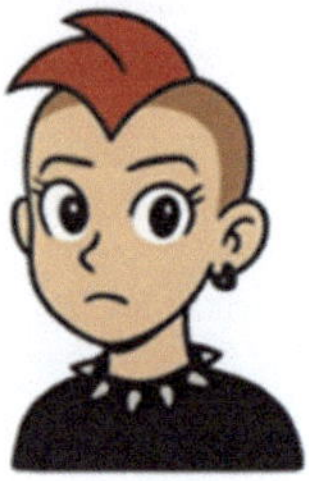

Did someone say something nice about you? Did someone compliment you?
List the positive comment here!

Fig. 9.5 (continued)

My Resources Portfolio

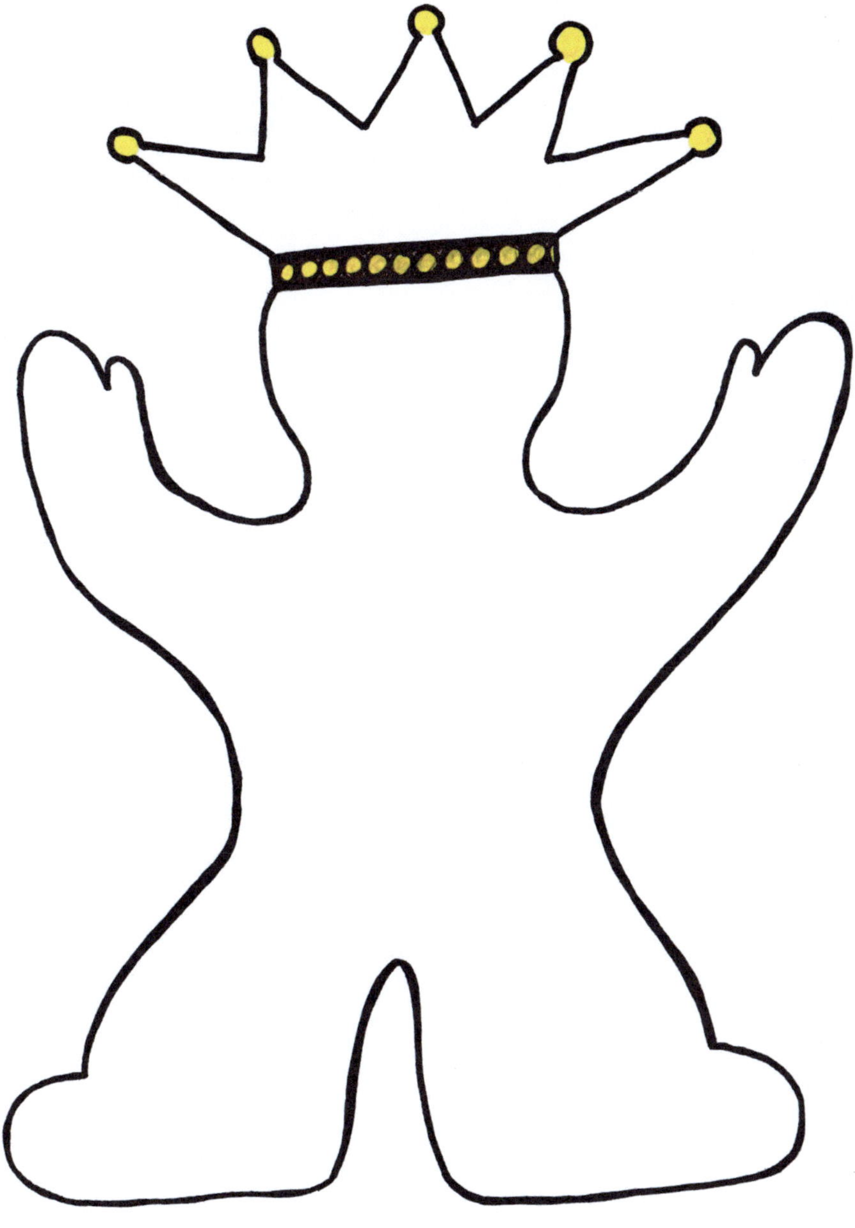

Fig. 9.5 (continued)

Positive Experiences

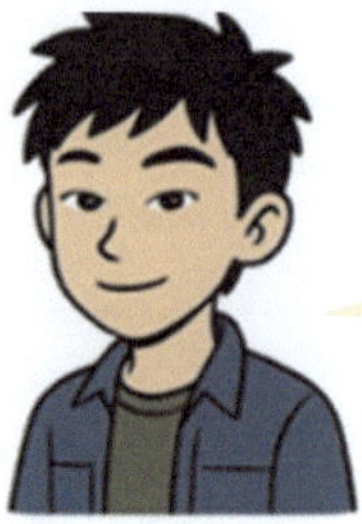

We experience positive moments every day. Even on a bad day, there are usually a few things to be happy about. Try to pay more attention to these positive moments and write down at least three every day. They don't have to be big events, look for small moments too. Moments such as getting a nice text message or someone cooking your favourite meal.

Monday

Tuesday

Wednesday

Fig. 9.5 (continued)

Positive Experiences

Thursday

Friday

Saturday

Sunday

Fig. 9.5 (continued)

Medication

10

There are no guidelines on pharmacological treatment for patients meeting CHR criteria. Meeting the CHR criteria by itself is not a reason for drug treatment. The recommendations published by the European Psychiatric Association (EPA) in 2015 focus on psychotherapy. Pharmacological approaches are not currently recommended but are the subject of research. In general, a very cautious approach to the use of antipsychotics is recommended. However, in cases of very high levels of distress due to CHR symptoms and loss of daily functioning, medication should be considered if psychotherapy is not sufficiently effective. A symptom-based approach is recommended. If positive symptoms are attenuated, low-dose treatment with an atypical antipsychotic may be considered. In clinical practice, it has proved useful to select the antipsychotic with the most tolerable side-effect profile for the patient. Medication should be monitored by an experienced psychiatrist. There are no data on how long pharmacotherapy should be continued for attenuated symptoms. As with the treatment of the first psychotic episode, it is advisable to continue medication for a prolonged period of time with complete freedom from symptoms. In any case, medication should not be stopped abruptly, and any attempt to stop should be closely monitored.

Antidepressants and omega-3 fatty acids have shown some evidence of a protective effect in randomized phase II studies. Adolescents meeting CHR criteria often suffer from comorbid psychiatric disorders, some of which can be treated with medication. For this reason, we have developed worksheets to increase compliance with medication. For the medication of comorbid symptoms, appropriate guidelines for drug treatment should be used.

Supplementary Information The online version contains supplementary material available at https://doi.org/10.1007/978-3-032-10341-3_10. The videos can be accessed individually by clicking the DOI link in the accompanying figure caption or by scanning this link with the SN More Media App.

N. Traber-Walker, M. Franscini, *Adolescents at Clinical High Risk for Psychosis*,
https://doi.org/10.1007/978-3-032-10341-3_10

Patients who make a transition to psychosis should be treated according to the current guidelines for the treatment of the first psychotic episode (e.g., S3 Deutsche Gesellschaft für Psychiatrie und Psychotherapie, Psychosomatik und Nervenheilkunde (DGPPN) or Schweizerische Gesellschaft für Psychiatrie und Psychotherapie (SGPP) treatment guidelines for schizophrenia). Pharmacotherapy with an antipsychotic is then an integral part of all current treatment recommendations. It should be noted, however, that adolescents generally have a more severe side-effect response to antipsychotics, and therefore the dose should be increased more slowly (start low–go slow). In the acute phase of the first psychotic episode, when the antipsychotic has not yet taken effect, adjunctive medication with a sedating anxiolytic may be very helpful.

Medication

The Robin Z app can be used to set medication reminders. Patients can record whether they have taken their medication in the logbook. In this way, the Robin app fulfills the function of a reminder and can also be used as a medication logbook. It makes sense to enter the medication into the app together with the patient during the therapy session. This makes it possible to check that the dose and time of administration have been recorded correctly.

There is a tutorial video "**Reminders**" (Fig. 10.1) for setting the medication reminder function.

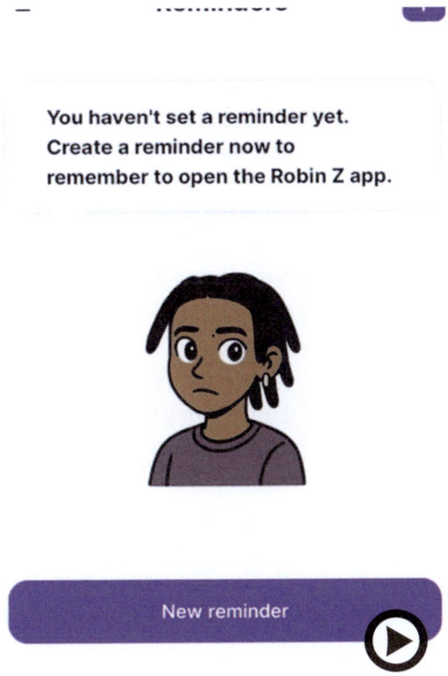
You haven't set a reminder yet.
Create a reminder now to
remember to open the Robin Z app.
New reminder

Fig. 10.1 Tutorial video "Reminders" (▶ https://doi.org/10.1007/000-k5s)

10.1 Providing Detailed Information About Effects and Side Effects

It is important that young people and their families are carefully informed about their medication. Not only should the biological mechanism of action of the medicine be discussed, but also the desired effect on the patient's state of mind and level of functioning.

Before starting medication, the fact that there are several products with different side-effect profiles should also be discussed. If the medication is not effective or the side effects are too severe, it may be advisable to change the medication.

Certain changes, such as tiredness, slowness, adynamia, or formal thinking problems, can be side effects of the medication as well as symptoms of psychotic development. Close monitoring is therefore essential.

It is strongly recommended that patients keep detailed records of their mood, symptoms, and possible (somatic) side effects when taking medication.

10.2 Compliance

Regular discussions about compliance are important. If symptoms improve or stop, adolescents may no longer see a reason to continue taking the medication. Out of a desire to be healthy, they may stop taking the medication every day, as the medication is seen as part of the illness. During the therapeutic sessions, it is therefore important to discuss with the adolescents, in a dialectical form, the relevance of continuing the medication. The worksheet "Pros and Cons" on the subject of medication can be helpful here.

Therapeutic Conversation Between the Therapist and Jo, a Teenager Who Has Been Treated with an Antipsychotic for 4 Months Due to Paranoid Schizophrenia

Jo:	I'm fine. The hallucinations are really over, and my current problems are related to the tablets. I've put on 7 kilos, I'm less able to do sport, and I can't party properly because I'm not allowed to drink alcohol.
Therapist:	I can absolutely see that. But let's look together at the positive effects of the medication.
Jo:	I have no more voices, but maybe they would have gone away on their own.
Therapist:	Let's remember what it was like before. How long have you had the voices?
Jo:	Uff... I think months, and I ended up hearing them every day.
Therapist:	Yeah, that's when you started the medication.
Jo:	And relatively soon the voices were no longer there.
Therapist:	What do you think? Is there a connection or not?
Jo:	Rather, yes.
Therapist:	The current state of medical research is that after a first episode of schizophrenia, you should take medication for at least a year to minimize the risk of relapse.
Jo:	Yes, I know that. They told me that when I started treatment.

Therapist:	However, I can understand that the side effects can be very distressing. Since the side effects you have reported are related to the dose of the medication, I suggest that we reduce the dose slightly. Then we can see if the side effects subside. This would mean that you would have to record the symptoms again, and we would have to see each other regularly every week. What do you think?
Jo:	Yes, OK for me.
Therapist:	The weight gain seems to be bothering you.
Jo:	Yes, I don't really feel good about my body... I haven't had a girlfriend for a long time.
Therapist:	We could consider three strategies: One, as discussed earlier, is to reduce the dose of the medication slightly. We should also discuss whether you are doing enough sport.
Jo:	Exactly, I get tired more quickly, and I'm less good at football, less coordinated. That's why I hardly play anymore.
Therapist:	I can understand that. But maybe there's something else you'd like to do now?
Jo:	I have a friend who uses a fitness app. Fifteen minutes a day.
Therapist:	I think it's a great idea. Could you imagine trying it before your next session?
Jo:	Yes, I could try it.
Therapist:	The third topic is food. Do you feel that you eat more than you used to?
Jo:	Yes, definitely. I eat more than I used to. Even between meals, I have more snacks and sweets.
Therapist:	That's where you could start, with snacking. Three main meals a day are important, and you shouldn't skip any of them.
Jo:	Maybe I could have just one snack during break instead of two?
Therapist:	Yes, that seems like a good plan with several small changes, but doable!

10.3 Worksheets

The following worksheets (Fig. 10.2) belong to this chapter and are available online for download in the context of the electronic chapter:

- Worksheet 53 "Biological Backgrounds".
- Worksheet 54 "Medication".
- Worksheet 55 "Pro/Con List".

Biological Background

In order for our brain cells to work well together, they send messages through messengers and receptors. One of these is messengers is called dopamine.

During a psychosis, there is an excess of dopamine.

The brain is in an abnormal state and sends the wrong signals. We can experience hallucinations and delusions as a result.

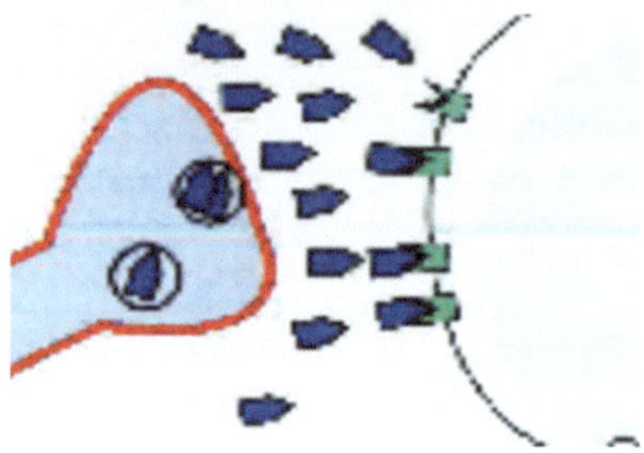

Brain cell **Dopamine** **Other brain cell**

How does medication work against psychosis?

Antipsychotic drugs work by preventing the oversupply of **Dopamine** that leads to overstimulation of the brain.

Since the receptors on the other cell are temporarily occupied by the drug, it takes up less of the excess dopamine. This leads to a reduction in psychotic symptoms. For the symptoms to disappear completely, the medication must be taken in the correct dosage for several months. The amount of medication and the duration of treatment are determined by the psychiatrist.

Medication

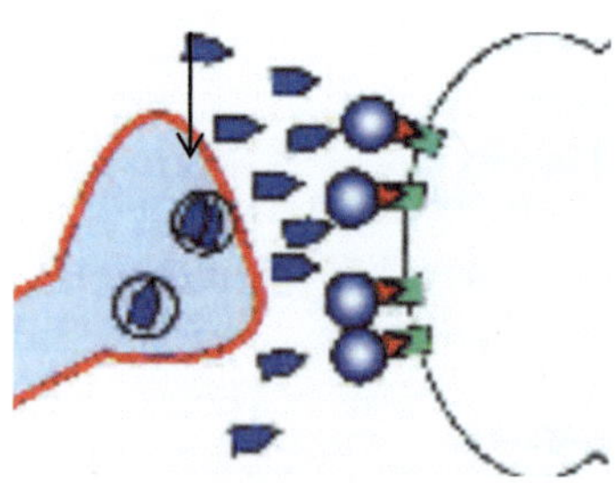

Brain cell **Dopamine** **Other brain cell**

Fig. 10.2 Worksheet 53 to Worksheet 55

Medication

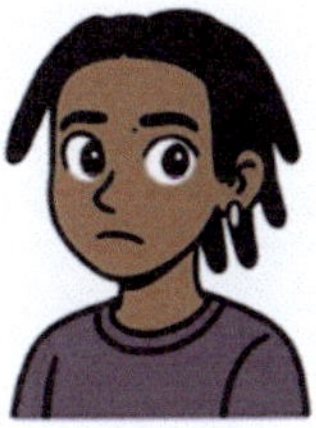

Medication needs to be taken regularly to be effective. Sometimes it can be difficult to remember to take your medication on time. Here are some ideas to help you remember to take your medication:

- Link taking your medication to another specific daily activity, such as always taking your medication with breakfast or always taking it when you brush your teeth in the evening.
- Use reminders, such as the reminder on your mobile phone or a small note next to your bed.
- Ask your parents to help you remember to take your medication.

Facts about the medication

✓ Find out about your medicines, how they work, and any side effects.

✓ If you have any questions during the week, make a note of them and discuss them with your therapist at your next appointment.

✓ Studies show that regular use of antipsychotic drugs reduces hallucinations and paranoia.

✓ Taking them regularly is associated with fewer relapses than taking them on an as-needed basis, for example, only when you have symptoms.

✓ If one medication does not work well, another may. It takes patience to find the right medication, especially at the beginning, because everyone reacts differently to medication. You need to find out which one works best for you.

✓ Medication should not be stopped suddenly as this can lead to withdrawal symptoms. If you want to stop taking your medication, talk to your doctor about it and make a plan to taper off slowly.

✓ Alcohol and medication do not mix well. You should avoid drinking alcohol as much as possible.

Fig. 10.2 (continued)

Pro/Con List

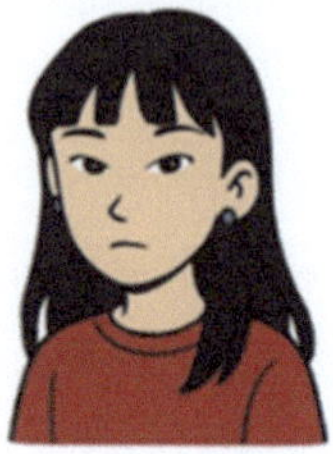

Sometimes you may not want to continue taking your medication. It is your right to decide if you want to continue taking it. Make a list of the advantages and disadvantages of the medication. It is important that you then discuss your thoughts and potential decision with your therapist before stopping your medication.

Advantages of medication	Disadvantages of medication

Fig. 10.2 (continued)

Further Reading

Amminger GP, Schäfer MR, Papageorgiou K, et al. Long-chain ω-3 fatty acids for indicated prevention of psychotic disorders: a randomised, placebo-controlled trial. Arch Gen Psychiatry. 2010;67(2):146–54. https://doi.org/10.1001/archgenpsychiatry.2009.192.

Bechdolf A, et al. PREVENT: a randomized controlled trial comparing cognitive behavioural therapy, clinical management and aripirazole and clinical management and placebo for the prevention of first episode psychosis. Early Interv Psychiatry. 2016;10:40.

Cornblatt BA, Lencz T, Smith CW, Olsen R, Auther AM, Nakayama E, et al. Can antidepressants be used to treat the schizophrenia prodrome? Results of a prospective, naturalistic treatment study of adolescents. J Clin Psychiatry. 2007;4:546–57.

Drzyzga ŁR, Marcinowska A, Obuchowicz E. Antiapoptotic and neurotrophic effects of antidepressants: a review of clinical and experimental studies. Brain Res Bull. 2009;79(5):248–57.

Fusar-Poli P, Valmaggia L, McGuire P. Can antidepressants prevent psychosis? Lancet. 2007;370(9601):1746–8.

McGorry PD, Nelson B, Markulev C, Yuen HP, Schäfer MR, Mossaheb N, et al. Effect of ω-3 polyunsaturated fatty acids in young people at ultrahigh risk for psychotic disorders: the NEURAPRO randomized clinical trial. JAMA psychiatry. 2017;74(1):19–27.

McGorry PD, Nelson B, Phillips LJ, Yuen HP, Francey SM, Thampi A, et al. Randomised controlled trial of interventions for young people at ultra-high risk of psychosis: twelve-month outcome. J Clin Psychiatry. 2013;74(4):349–56.

Pagsberg AK, Jeppesen P, Klauber DG, Jensen KG, Rudå D, Stentebjerg-Olesen M, et al. Quetiapine extended release versus aripiprazole in children and adolescents with first-episode psychosis: the multicentre, double-blind, randomised tolerability and efficacy of antipsychotics (TEA) trial. Lancet Psychiatry. 2017;4(8):605–18.

Yung AR, Phillips LJ, Nelson B, Francey SM, Yuen HP, Simmons MB, et al. Randomised controlled trial of interventions for young people at ultra high risk for psychosis: 6-month analysis. J Clin Psychiatry. 2011;72(4):430.

Ruhrmann S, et al. Acute effects of treatment for prodromal symptoms for people putatively in a late initial prodromal state of psychosis. Br J Psychiatry. 2007;191(S51):s88–95.

Samara MT, Leucht C, Leeflang MM, Anghelescu IG, Chung YC, Crespo-Facorro B, et al. Early improvement as a predictor of later response to antipsychotics in schizophrenia: a diagnostic test review. Am J Psychiatry. 2015;172(7):617–29.

Schmidt SJ, Schultze-Lutter F, Schimmelmann BG, Maric NP, Salokangas RKR, Riecher-Rössler A, et al. EPA guidance on the early intervention in clinical high risk states of psychoses. Eur Psychiatry. 2015;30(3):388–404.

Maintaining Stability

11

11.1 Problem-Solving Strategies

Adolescents with CHR symptoms often feel overwhelmed by everyday stressors, and subjectively perceived excessive levels of stress can also lead to the onset of psychosis. Strengthening the ability to cope with stress is therefore a major objective of therapy.

As it is not in the therapist's power to reduce all the stress in the patient's life, it is important to work on individual strategies for coping with stress.

The problem-solving worksheets provide patients with a possible strategy for coping with challenging situations in everyday life. The first worksheet provides a nine-point problem-solving approach.

- What is the problem?
- How have I solved similar problems in the past?
- What helped?
- What was not helpful?
- What possible solutions do I see (whether realistic or not)?
- Evaluate and compare possible solutions.
- Choose the best possible solution.
- How can this solution be implemented?
- Which of my resources can help me solve the problem?
- Are there other people I can involve in the solution?
- What small steps are needed to achieve my solution?
- Realizing the solution.

Supplementary Information The online version contains supplementary material available at https://doi.org/10.1007/978-3-032-10341-3_11. The videos can be accessed individually by clicking the DOI link in the accompanying figure caption or by scanning this link with the SN More Media App.

N. Traber-Walker, M. Franscini, *Adolescents at Clinical High Risk for Psychosis*,
https://doi.org/10.1007/978-3-032-10341-3_11

The problem-solving approach should be explained in detail during treatment so that patients can use it in their daily lives. An example from the patient's life can be used to illustrate the model.

The first step is to encourage patients to think about how they coped with similar difficulties in the past and what they found helpful. This automatically recalls and activates existing coping strategies. At the same time, without the therapist having to mention it, these earlier coping experiences illustrate that problems are a part of life and that tools can be acquired from them. The second worksheet, "Problem Solving Ideas," is about brainstorming solutions. All solutions that come to the patient's mind should be written down. The advantages and disadvantages of the solutions are then identified and used to rank the solutions in the last column.

If patients decide on a particular solution, this solution should be organized into different steps (see worksheet "Solution Implementation"). Again, it is important that patients think carefully about how to carry out each step. For each step, they should consider which of their skills might be needed in order to carry out that specific step. This will remind them of the strengths they possess that can help them overcome problems.

When working with this schema, the therapist should point out that there are several possible solutions. Even if the (supposedly) best solution does not work, the patient should not give up; continue to try the second or third best option.

11.2 Crisis Management

The term 'crisis' does not mean the same thing to everyone. For many people meeting CHR criteria, a crisis means that their symptoms become more severe, or they experience more CHR symptoms, which can increase anxiety. Suicidal thoughts are another issue that can lead to a crisis. Suicidal thoughts are reported by many people with CHR. Treatment manuals for adults often recommend that crises be clearly defined and that a crisis plan be activated. However, our clinical experience of working with adolescents shows that it is better not to define crises too narrowly. Adolescents' symptoms can change very quickly, and they may suddenly experience new symptoms that were not anticipated and, therefore, were not defined as a crisis in advance. This may also be the case with suicidal thoughts. Although the crisis plan is usually drawn up in relation to a specific scenario, it should also be designed so that the strategy can be used in any other possible crisis situation. As the topic of crisis is often raised during the initial consultation, the preparation of a detailed crisis plan is often one of the first steps in therapy or even the first thing to be done during the diagnostic phase.

- **Crisis Plan:** The Robin Z app has a feature for crisis situations. The users can enter and save their crisis plan. This means that they always have it with them and can refer to it whenever they are in an emergency situation.
- **Emergency Contacts:** Emergency contacts can also be saved in the crisis plan and called directly from the app if necessary. This has the advantage that in a crisis situation, patients don't have to look up a phone number from the addresses. Calls are made via the mobile operator's normal network.

Information on the crisis plan in Robin Z can be found in the tutorial video "**Crisis Plan**" (Fig. 11.1).

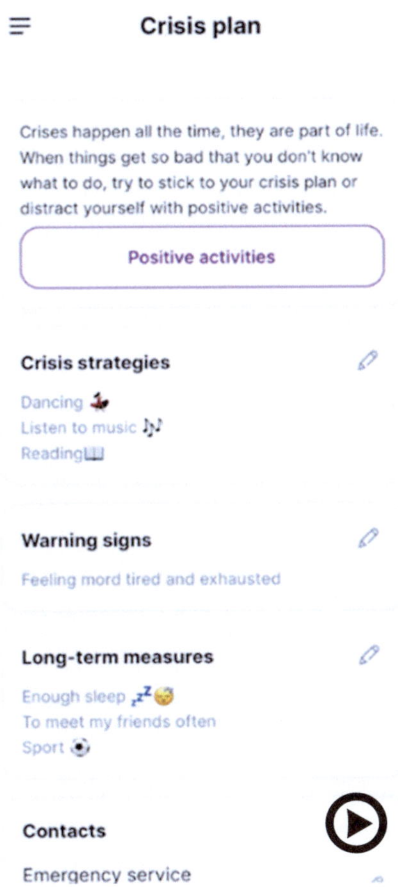

Fig. 11.1 Tutorial video "Crisis plan" (▶ https://doi.org/10.1007/000-k5t)

The risk of self-harm or harm towards others needs to be explored in detail during the first contact. If the first contact takes place in the presence of parents, it is important to talk to the adolescent again privately about suicidal thoughts and endangering others, as many adolescents do not want to speak of such things in the presence of their parents. It is important to take all indications of suicidal tendencies seriously without being catastrophic. Instead, clear agreements should be made about how to deal with situations involving suicidal thoughts. The same applies, of course, to thoughts of harming others.

Therapists are often faced with the dilemma of patient confidentiality when it comes to self-harm or harm to others. Feedback to parents is very important. However, some young patients do not want their parents to know about these thoughts. It is important not to ignore their wishes but to explore the reasons for their concerns. Adolescents often don't want to burden their parents. Otherwise, they may be afraid that their parents will overreact. Together, it should be discussed what can be told to the parents and how. In retrospect, patients usually find it a relief when their parents are informed. Our clinical practice also shows that parents usually react more appropriately than their children had expected.

Both parents and their children should be made aware of the 24-hour helpline and encouraged to call in the event of a crisis. Experience shows that the majority of patients will only call in a crisis. If, in individual cases, calls become more frequent and the number is used as a kind of helpline outside of therapy appointments, this needs to be discussed with the patient. In such cases, clear agreements should be made about when to call the emergency services and when not to call.

The long-term goal of therapy in regard to self-efficacy is to enable young people to manage crises themselves without relying on emergency services. The therapy sessions can be used to discuss coping strategies for a crisis situation and to define appropriate strategies that can be written down in the crisis plan. In our consultations, it has proven useful to ask patients to think of a total of three activities they would like to do to calm themselves in the event of a crisis. They should spend at least fifteen minutes on the first activity. If they do not feel better after the first activity, they should continue with the second activity for at least another fifteen minutes and, if necessary, try the third activity after a further fifteen minutes.

When choosing activities for the crisis plan, the therapist should ensure that the activities are not too dependent on time and place. It does not make much sense to say "I'll go riding in a crisis" if the horse is stationed five kilometers away and can only be ridden twice a week. On the other hand, if the patient has their own horse around the corner, then riding may be an option. The therapist should also consider at least one activity that can be done at night. Quiet activities such as watching television, surfing the Internet, or listening to music are appropriate.

If, after all three activities, the patient still feels as bad as before, it should be agreed that an adult should be informed. The therapist must insist that an adult carer be the emergency contact. Siblings or friends should not be burdened with the crisis. Usually, there is agreement that, in an emergency, the patient will inform the parents or, if this is not possible, the emergency services.

In addition to acute crisis strategies and emergency contacts, the worksheet "Crisis Plan" includes warning signs. Patients are encouraged to list warning signs that may alert them to an upcoming crisis, even before the acute crisis occurs.

The final part of the crisis plan is long-term measures. Together, the patient and therapist should consider how the patient can prevent crises in the future. What will help them feel stable over time? This could include healthy everyday habits such as regular meals, regular physical activity, or getting enough sleep. Long-term goals should also be listed here, such as a planned trip, special events the patient is looking forward to, or plans for the longer term, such as going to university or moving away from home.

Therapeutic Conversation with Michael

Michael has been suffering from suicidal thoughts recently. He does not actually want to hurt himself, but the thoughts can sometimes be very intense and overwhelming. The following emergency procedure is agreed upon with Michael:

Therapist:	What helps you in these moments? How do you distract yourself?
Michael:	It works best when I go out and meet friends. But that's not always possible. Especially late in the evening when I'm at home and should be in bed.
Therapist:	Do you manage to fall asleep despite these thoughts?
Michael:	Rarely. I usually get very restless and can barely stay in bed.
Therapist:	What do you do then?
Michael:	Sometimes I take a shower. It distracts me and relaxes me a bit.
Therapist:	Very good, that's a very good strategy. We could use that as the first activity in the crisis plan. What do you think?
Michael:	(nods) I think it's good, yes.
Therapist:	Do your thoughts always go away when you have a shower?
Michael:	No, sometimes not.
Therapist:	What could you do then? As a next step?
Michael:	Sometimes it helps to write with friends.
Therapist:	That's a good idea, but what if your friends don't reply? Or do they always reply?
Michael:	No, sometimes they don't see the message; they're asleep or something. But it's even worse when they read my message and don't reply right away. Then I feel really bad.
Therapist:	That's why I asked. I think chatting with friends is a good idea, but sometimes it's just not possible. What could you do instead that would also cheer you up?
Michael:	There are certain TikTok videos that I always find funny. There's this one guy who makes me laugh almost every time I watch him. No matter how bad I feel.
Therapist:	I think that's a very good plan. How about "watching TikTok videos with this guy" as your next activity?
Michael:	Yeah, I like that.
Therapist:	So that would be the second step if showering doesn't help: Watch videos for at least 15 minutes. What could you do as a third activity if you still have these thoughts?
Michael:	Well, smoking often helps. But I can't go out on the balcony late at night because my parents can hear me, and they don't want me smoking late at night.
Therapist:	It's important that it's an activity you can do all the time, not just in certain circumstances. What else might help you?
Michael:	Listening to the music of my favorite band often makes me feel better.

Therapist:	Great, so your third activity is listening to your favorite band. For at least 15 minutes. But what do you think? Could this plan really help, or is there a chance that the thoughts will still be there after all three activities?
Michael:	I actually think that these activities will help me.
Therapist:	Me too. However, it's important that we talk hypothetically about what you do if the suicidal thoughts don't get better or even get worse despite these three steps. I clearly heard you say earlier that you don't want to hurt yourself and that you really do want to go on living.
Michael:	Yes, I don't really want to die.
Therapist:	Can we make a clear agreement that no matter how strong the thoughts get, you won't do anything regrettable without first trying the activities from the crisis plan?
Michael:	(nods) yeah, I think that's good.
Therapist:	It's just that sometimes you may feel so bad that all these activities don't help enough. I don't want anything to happen to you. Can you imagine calling us if you don't feel better? To our emergency service?
Michael:	Yes, maybe. Hm. we can agree on that, yes.
Therapist:	This is a very important point for me. I know it's not easy to call here. I want you to be completely honest. Can you imagine calling our emergency service when you're so unwell that you don't want to live?
Michael:	Well, I don't really know...
Therapist:	A lot of young people find it difficult to call here. I can understand that. Why do you think it is difficult for you?
Michael:	I don't know the person on the phone. It's not you.
Therapist:	No, it's not me, you're right. It will be someone else who also works here. A doctor who is also bound by patient confidentiality and whose job it is to help young people in crisis.
Michael:	So what do I say on the phone? "Hello, I'm Michael, and I want to kill myself."
Therapist:	(nods) you can say exactly that.
Michael:	But then I feel really stupid.
Therapist:	I can understand that. Other teenagers say the same thing. But you know, this person on the phone expects people to say things like that when they call here. Nobody calls here in the middle of the night to talk about the weather or to order a pizza. Instead, when the phone rings, the emergency service clearly assumes that the person calling is not feeling well. The idea of talking to a stranger on the phone about your suicidal thoughts may sound strange to you. But that stranger hears these things all the time. It's their job.
Michael:	I hadn't thought of it that way.
Therapist:	That's why we're talking about it. Now that you think about it, could you imagine calling here in an emergency?
Michael:	Yes, I would.
Therapist:	Do you still have concerns?
Michael:	I'm still not comfortable calling them. But you're right, that's what this number is for.
Therapist:	It's very, very important to me that I can rely on you to call here in an emergency.
Michael:	Yeah, it's OK.
Therapist:	Very good. Is it OK if we enter the crisis plan directly into the app on your mobile phone? And store the phone number of our emergency service there?
Michael:	Yes, I can do that.

11.3 Recognizing Early Warning Signs

Most psychotherapy patients feel better after a few months and see their symptoms decline. It is useful to discuss with patients what, in retrospect, they consider to be their early warning signs and how they would recognize them if they were beginning to feel worse again. This can be documented on the "My Early Warning Signs" worksheet. At the same time, the patient and therapist should think together about how to deal with the early warning signs. The first step is to be aware of these signs. Keeping a mood and symptom diary or continuing to use the logbook in the app Robin Z is a good way to do this. A single occurrence of one of the early warning signs does not necessarily mean that the next crisis is imminent. If the warning signs persist, the first step might be to intensify the coping strategies learned in therapy and thereby reduce the individual symptoms. At the same time, it may be helpful to consider whether there is a specific reason why the warning signs are occurring now. Is there a particular stressor? As stress often plays an important role in triggering symptoms, it is useful to consider strategies to reduce current stress levels.

Therapeutic Conversation with Lucy

Therapist:	I'm very glad to hear, Lucy, that you've been feeling better for a while now.
Lucy:	It's hard to believe how my life has turned around. I'm getting better grades, I'm seeing my friends more often, and I'm having far fewer arguments with my family. I just hope it stays that way.
Therapist:	We have often talked about how crises and difficult times are part of life. You can't always prevent them. The good thing is that you have overcome a really difficult episode.
Lucy:	Well, I still hope that I will never feel as bad as I did then.
Therapist:	Of course. I wish you the same. We've talked before about how an episode like this doesn't start overnight but develops over a period of time. The earlier you recognize the signs of a possible new onset, the better you can avoid a new episode with difficult symptoms. Mental health problems are similar to physical health problems. If you take it easy when you have a mild cold, you can sometimes avoid getting the flu. That's why I'd like you to write a list of early warning signs. What do you think?
Lucy:	(nods) yes, absolutely.
Therapist:	If you think back to the time when you were so unwell. What would you say were the very first signs from your point of view? The first changes?
Lucy:	Well, I would say the changes in my mood. I was less happy, more tired, and exhausted. In addition, everything was becoming too much for me. I found my class too loud, the voices in the playground, and the music in the background. Everything was too loud for me. Suddenly, the others started to bother me. I never had such thoughts before; I always enjoyed being around people and loved breaks.
Therapist:	What is it like now?
Lucy:	I no longer have a problem with it. Only very rarely, perhaps when I've slept badly, do I tolerate all these stimuli around me a little less.
Therapist:	I think that's a very good observation on your part. It was all too much for you at the time, and you could not cope with all the sensory input around you. We've all had days like that. When we lack sleep, when we feel slightly ill, or just like that, there are days when we can take less. It only gets difficult when it happens every day for a long time.

Lucy:	(nods) yes, it got worse and worse.
Therapist:	So this could be an important warning sign for you. What would you call it?
Lucy:	Hypersensitivity.
Therapist:	And it is quite normal to feel hypersensitivity, as you say, in many situations. So we would only call it an early warning sign if it lasted for several weeks. I'd say at least two weeks.
Lucy:	Every day?
Therapist:	At least almost every day. Does that make sense to you? The point is not to immediately fear the worst, but to first observe such an early warning sign.
Lucy:	Yes, that's good.
Therapist:	That is why I always advise my patients to record their symptoms. This means that for at least two weeks, you should keep a close eye on your mood and sensitivity, checking them several times a day. I would also advise you to keep track of your sleep and your ability to concentrate. It is best to make a note of the situations in which your hypersensitivity is particularly strong.
Lucy:	So that I can see if there is a specific reason for it?
Therapist:	Exactly. These early warning signs usually appear when we are going through a stressful time.
Lucy:	Yes, it's true. Just before the last holidays, it happened again. We had a lot of exams and then the dance project. Even though I was feeling much better and had hardly any symptoms, I was much more sensitive again. Everything was too much for me. I was really exhausted in the evenings, and sometimes at dinner, I hardly felt like talking to my family. As soon as the exams were over and I was on holiday, things got better.
Therapist:	You have observed this very well. That's why the first step, if you're experiencing the early warning signs again, is to think about what strategies might be helpful to reduce your current stress levels.
Lucy:	OK, but what do I do if this hypersensitivity persists?
Therapist:	What do you think might be useful at that point?
Lucy:	Hm, I'm not sure. I used to withdraw a lot. For example, at school, I used to spend the breaks in the classroom instead of spending them with friends.
Therapist:	And did that help?
Lucy:	At first, but as time went on, it got worse because of the withdrawal.
Therapist:	We've talked about this before—Sometimes it makes sense to withdraw.
Lucy:	But not always!
Therapist:	What could you do instead if you felt that things were getting too much for you?
Lucy:	Maybe I could ask a friend to go for a walk in a quiet place. So we're not in the middle of the crowd. Then I'll have a bit of time to recover, but I won't be alone.
Therapist:	I think that's a very good idea. It could certainly be helpful at that moment.

11.4 Adjusting the Frequency of Therapy Sessions

Treatment should not be continued longer than necessary. Once the patient feels stable, treatment should be reduced gradually. Once the initial acute phase is over, symptoms have subsided, and the patient has made progress in coping with stress and managing symptoms, treatment intervals can be increased to two weeks. This is advisable for two reasons:

- It shows patients that they can manage without therapy for a week. In terms of helping people to help themselves, the therapist should prevent patients from becoming dependent on therapy.
- Adolescents, in particular, are more likely to stay motivated if they don't have weekly therapy appointments on top of their many other commitments. Over time, the appointments can be reduced to monthly meetings.

The most important thing is to meet the patients' needs. Are they ready to change the frequency of their sessions, or do they still need their weekly appointment? However, to avoid dependency, lower frequencies are encouraged.

Therapeutic Conversation with Michael

Michael:	If I'm honest, I don't think it's a good idea for me to go a whole month without a session.
Therapist:	I'm glad you're being so honest. Tell me what you're worried about.
Michael:	Well, a month is a long time. A lot can happen. A whole month without therapy? We've never done that before.
Therapist:	That's right, the longest we've gone was two weeks, and that went really well. A month is not much longer.
Michael:	Hm...
Therapist:	You do not seem convinced. In other words, what would have to happen for you to imagine coming only once a month?
Michael:	Well, I have to be absolutely sure that it won't get worse again. That I won't have a relapse.
Therapist:	Is there such a thing? A guarantee against relapse?
Michael:	Unfortunately, no. that's why I say...
Therapist:	If we meet every two weeks, will that prevent you from relapsing?
Michael:	I think it will.
Therapist:	Why is that?
Michael:	I don't know, I just feel better. You would probably notice if I got worse again.

Therapist:	Do you think I would notice before you? In that one hour every two weeks? Or before your parents, your friends, or someone else close to you? Someone who sees you almost every day?
Michael:	Well, you're the expert. You can judge the situation better than I can.
Therapist:	Actually, I see it differently. I think you are still the expert when it comes to yourself. Then there are the people closest to you, who see you almost every day. Even when I do see you, I only see you for one hour. In that hour, I rely on your input. You tell me what's going on with you. As we discussed, I can't read minds any more than anyone else.
Michael:	That's true, but I feel more confident when I come to our regular sessions.
Therapist:	I think I understand what you're saying. I just don't think that coming here once a week is going to prevent you from having another crisis.
Michael:	I just don't want to go through another year like last year.
Therapist:	I can understand that, Michael. You have managed to get through such a difficult time. Everything you have learned so far, in therapy and elsewhere, will be available to you the next time something happens. Now you have different skills to deal with mood swings or any possible symptoms than you did before.
Michael:	That's right.
Therapist:	Of course, you can also contact me immediately if you feel that you are no longer feeling well. You can always make an appointment. You don't have to wait four weeks. What do you think, Michael, would you be prepared to try a break from therapy?

What to Do If Patients Are Reluctant to Decrease the Frequency of Therapy?
When it is time to decrease the frequency of therapy sessions, some patients will feel reluctant. The therapist should identify the reasons for such hesitancies with the patient during the session. Concerns are often raised, which can then be addressed in therapy. Many patients say that regular appointments make them feel more secure that their symptoms will not worsen. This needs to be discussed openly, noting that even with weekly sessions, symptoms can worsen. People do not usually become psychotic from one day to the next. A deterioration can also be seen if the patient only attends fortnightly or monthly sessions. Of course, the frequency can be increased at any time if necessary.

What Should I Do If Patients Want to Stop Treatment Too Quickly?
Sometimes, motivation for therapy decreases as symptoms improve, though the therapist still feels that the patient needs to continue with regular sessions. However, if the patient wants to stop therapy, the therapist should accept this. It is recommended that the reasons for this be discussed. Arrangements can be made with the adolescent to attend follow-up sessions at longer intervals. In addition, the list of early warning signs could be used to determine the circumstances under which the frequency of sessions should be increased again.

Full recovery is not a prerequisite for stopping treatment. Instead, a treatment period can be completed when the patient has stabilized, and progress is possible. A positive experience is essential. Without a positive experience in therapy, patients may be discouraged from seeking help in the event of another crisis.

11.5 Treatment Termination

In the final session, the progress of the treatment should be discussed in detail. It can be useful to have the patients themselves write down their progress and reflect on what helped them get there. The last two worksheets, "How Do I Maintain Stability?" and "Letter to the Future Me," are suitable for this. The worksheet "How Do I Maintain Stability?" allows the patient and therapist to write down helpful behaviors and strategies learned during therapy. The "Letter to the Future Me," on the other hand, is a very personal letter from the patient to the future self, which the therapist does not necessarily have to read. It should be up to the patient to decide whether or not to share it with the therapist. The aim is for them to write an encouraging letter to their future self for possible future crises or episodes with symptoms.

After treatment, it is advisable to have follow-up examinations to detect any changes in CHR symptoms. In our service, we typically offer three follow-up visits within the first two years, with the first follow-up visit taking place six months after the end of treatment. At the follow-up appointments, the patient's current health status, the presence of CHR symptoms, and any changes in their general life situation since the last appointment are explored. If there has been a negative progression, a follow-up visit offers the opportunity to start a new treatment period, and a change of therapist can be considered. For patients who no longer report symptoms, it is recommended that follow-up visits highlight positive changes and progress. The materials in Chap. 9 are particularly suitable for this purpose. For example, new ideas can be added to the list of strengths or the "My Resources Portfolio" during the follow-up meeting. The original goals can also be revisited. Patients are often unaware that they are at a completely different point, and comparing their current situation with the initial situation can be motivating.

Therapeutic Conversation with Michael

Michael:	It is very strange to think that today is the last time I will have a session with you.
Therapist:	Yes, you have been coming for regular sessions for almost a year. When we think of what you've achieved in that time, wow! You really are at a very different place in your life.
Michael:	When I first came here, I felt so bad. I never thought I would be able to get out of that mess.
Therapist:	I took another look at your previous therapy goals. Look at the list. What do you think when you look at it?
Michael:	Wow, I didn't even remember that. I can really say with confidence that I've achieved them all.
Therapist:	I would say the same. What do you think? Should we write down all the positive changes together?
Michael:	I don't know, maybe we could. Yeah.
Therapist:	Where were you a year ago? And where are you today?
Michael:	I still have my apprenticeship. This is my last year before graduation, and it looks like I'll be able to complete it.
Therapist:	That is certainly an important achievement.

Michael:	I'm socializing more with my friends again. I've also managed to distance myself from so-called friends who weren't friends at all. I may have a smaller circle of friends now, but the ones I do have are really good friends. I trust them.
Therapist:	I think that's a meaningful change. Your friendships have increased in quality!
Michael:	Yes, you could say that.
Therapist:	What else? What else have you achieved?
Michael:	Well, I stopped hearing voices months ago. And my mood is more stable. I'm happier and more content.
Therapist:	When you think back now, what advice would you give Michael from back then?
Michael:	Stay active. I withdrew a lot back then. I often lie in bed, doing nothing or sleeping during the day. That didn't do me any good at all.
Therapist:	Yes, I think that's an important point. What else would you recommend to yourself?
Michael:	No matter how stressful my day has been and no matter how much I have to do, I should spend some time on enjoyable activities.
Therapist nods:	Any other advice?
Michael:	One important thing I've learned in therapy is that I don't have to deal with my difficulties alone. It's OK to get help.
Therapist:	I'm glad to hear that. Of course I agree. Is there anything else you would like to say to Michael from that time?
Michael:	I would say it's just a phase. A difficult phase with many crises, but it is only temporary. There will be a better time after that.

11.6 Worksheets

The following worksheets (Fig. 11.2) belong to this chapter and are available online for download in the context of the electronic chapter:

· Worksheet 56 "Problem-Solving Approach".
· Worksheet 57 "Problem Solving Ideas".
· Worksheet 58 "Solution Implementation".
· Worksheet 59 "Crisis Plan".
· Worksheet 60 "My Early Warning Signs".
· Worksheet 61 "Maintain Stability".
· Worksheet 62 "Letter to the Future Me".

Poblem-Solving Approach

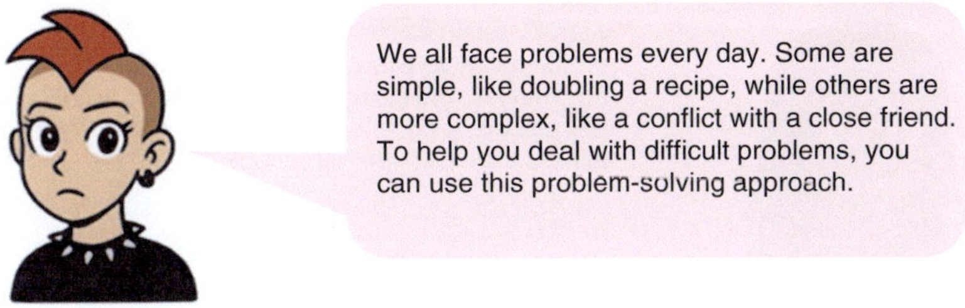

Problem-solving approach:

1. What is the problem?
2. How have I solved similar problems in the past?
3. In the past, what helped?
4. In the past, what was not helpful?
5. What possible solutions do I see (whether realistic or not)?
6. Evaluate and compare possible solutions.
7. Choose the best possible solution.
8. How can this solution be implemented?

a) Which of my resources can I use to solve the problem?

b) Are there helpers, other people I can involve?

c) What small steps are needed?

9. Realising the solution

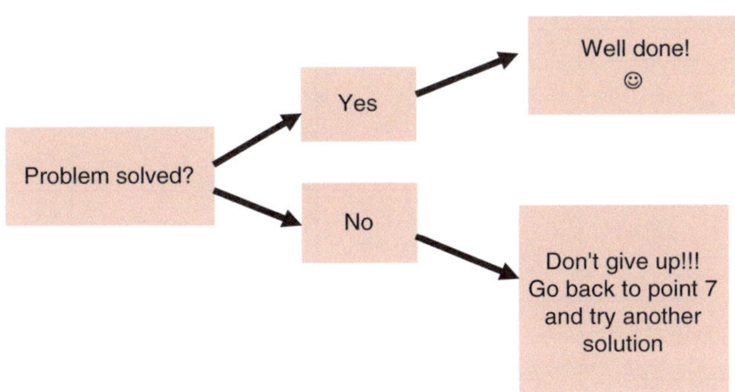

Fig. 11.2 Worksheet 56 to Worksheet 62

Problem Solving Ideas

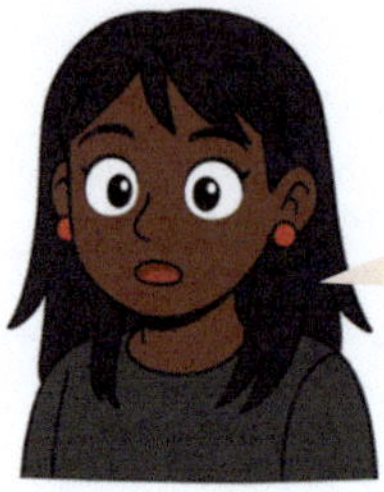

Start by listing all the possible solutions to the problem that you can think of. Then outline the advantages and disadvantages of each option. In the last column, evaluate and rate which solution you think is the most effective.

Solution	Advantages	Disadvantages	Ranking

Fig. 11.2 (continued)

Solution Implementation

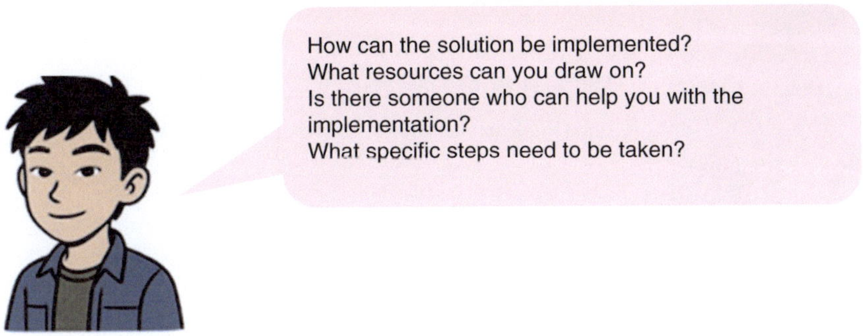

Key steps in the solution process	My resources	Who can help me with this?	Done

Fig. 11.2 (continued)

Crisis Plan

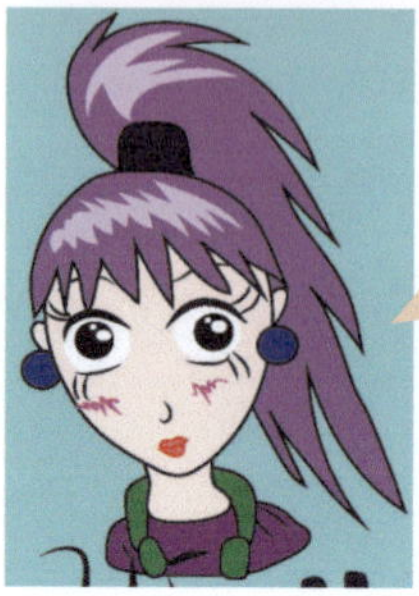

Crises happen all the time, they are part of life. When things get so bad that you

don't know what to do, try to stick to your crisis plan.

1. Crisis strategies: What makes you feel better in an acute crisis?

2. Warning signs: What are the first signs that you're getting worse?

3. Long-term measures: What could help you feel better in the long term?

If you're still not feeling better:

Let your parents know or call the following emergency number:

Fig. 11.2 (continued)

My Early Warning Signs

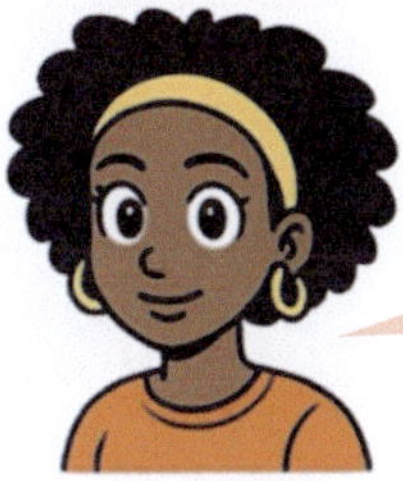

What are your personal early warning signs that you are getting worse? If you are able to recognise these early signs, you can do something to prevent the situation from getting worse.

My early warning sign	What I can do about it

Fig. 11.2 (continued)

Maintain Stability

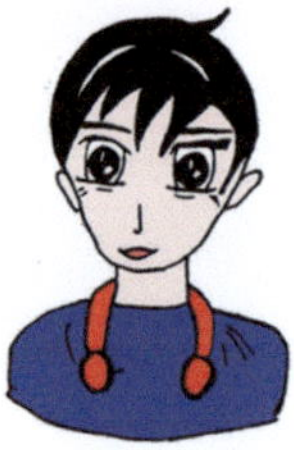

What do you think you can do to stay well?
What strategies can help you maintain stability?
What activities are good for you?
How can you react when things suddenly become too much for you?
Collect tips from yourself and list them here.

Fig. 11.2 (continued)

Letter to the Future

Fig. 11.2 (continued)

MIX
Papier aus verantwortungsvollen Quellen
Paper from responsible sources
FSC® C105338

If you have any concerns about our products,
you can contact us on
ProductSafety@springernature.com

In case Publisher is established outside the EU,
the EU authorized representative is:
Springer Nature Customer Service Center GmbH
Europaplatz 3, 69115 Heidelberg, Germany

Printed by Libri Plureos GmbH
in Hamburg, Germany